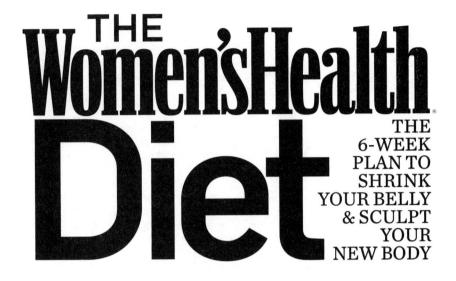

THE
Women'sHealth
Diet

THE 6-WEEK PLAN TO SHRINK YOUR BELLY & SCULPT YOUR NEW BODY

STEPHEN PERRINE
with LEAH FLICKINGER and
the EDITORS of *Women's Health*

RODALE

© 2011 by Rodale Inc.

All rights reserved. No part of this publication may be reproduced or t ransmitted in any form or by any means, electronic or mechanical, including photocopying, recording, or any other information storage and retrieval system, without the written permission of the publisher.

Rodale books may be purchased for business or promotional use or for special sales. For information, please write to:

Special Markets Department, Rodale Inc.,
733 Third Avenue, New York, NY 10017

Women's Health is a registered trademark of Rodale Inc.

Printed in the United States of America

Rodale Inc. makes every effort to use acid-free ♾, recycled paper ♻.

Book design by the Men's Health and Women's Health
Branded Books design team:
Mark Michaelson, Elizabeth Neal, Laura White, and Mike Smith,
with George Karabotsos
Interior photos by Mitch Mandell
Hair and makeup by Colleen Kobrick

Cover design by Joe Heroun / Cover photo by Beth Bischoff

Library of Congress Cataloging-in-Publication Data is on file with the publisher.

ISBN-13: 978-1-60961-038-8

4 6 8 10 9 7 5 3   hardcover

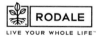

We inspire and enable people to improve their lives and the world around them.

For Jennifer

CONTENTS

FOREWORD

If you're a reader of *Women's Health,*
then you already know that my team of editors and I are obsessed
with helping women reach their fitness, weight loss, and nutrition
goals. Every month, we scour the latest studies in prestigious
journals, interview dozens of the country's top experts, and, most
important, we actually practice what they preach—in the gym, in
the kitchen, even in the office—so that we can serve as guinea pigs
before passing their tips on to you. Our task—no, our mission—is to
deliver the most authoritative, evidence-based advice on how to
look and feel your best. We're not interested in fads and gimmicks
that might work in the short term but set you up for failure in the
long run. We're interested in results. And over the last decade,
we've learned a thing or two about what works and what doesn't
when you want to lose weight and feel great.

We've learned that starvation only backfires, that you need enough of the right foods—and at the right times—to turn your body into a lean, flab-fighting machine. (And instead of counting calories, you simply follow seven simple rules for eating that we call the Secrets of the Slim.) We've learned that grueling workouts can discourage rather than motivate, and that you only need to exercise three times a week for 30 minutes a day to shed fat and sculpt and tone your body. And we've learned that limiting yourself to bland, boring foods just isn't necessary—you can eat at chain restaurants from Red Lobster to White Castle and stay slim (provided you pick from our list of the 250 Best Foods for Women.)

The Women's Health Diet takes all our research and experience and distills it into one simple program. Because here's what else we've learned: Women are incredibly industrious and busy creatures. Between demanding jobs and family and significant others, we can barely get to the grocery store much less embark on an all-consuming new fitness regime. Above all other considerations, the *Women's Health* Diet was designed to be pragmatic—to give you real results instead of pie-in-the-sky hypotheticals. That's why we put the *Women's Health* Diet to the test first with a group of women with a variety of goals. Some wanted to lose weight, some wanted to firm up, some wanted a flat belly—but the fact that they were all able to reach their targets speaks to the reliability and versatility of this program.

I'm pleased and proud to introduce you to the *Women's Health* Diet. Consider it your ultimate guide to getting the body you've always wanted. Because after all, it's good to be you.

Michele Promaulayko
Editor-in-Chief
Women's Health

ACKNOWLEDGMENTS

One summer's day in 1991, while taking out the recycling, I glanced down at the newspaper and saw an advertisement for a junior-level job at a new magazine called *Men's Health*, the brother publication of a future publishing powerhouse called *Women's Health*. I drove my family out to Emmaus, Pennsylvania, to apply.

I didn't get that job.

Luckily, another position opened up soon after, and from that moment on, I've been fortunate to work with the greatest team of journalists, publishers, and health-care professionals ever assembled. In particular:

Maria Rodale and the Rodale family, who have been fighting to awaken us to the connection between our health and our environment for more than 60 years. I hope this book brings readers one step closer to realizing a healthier future.

David Zinczenko, whose support, encouragement, and grace under pressure have made possible my endeavors, and those of many others, at Rodale Inc.

Michele Promaulayko, under whose leadership *Women's Health* has blossomed into an extraordinary magazine adventure.

My brilliant co-author, Leah Flickinger.

George Karabotsos, Debbie McHugh, Laura White, Mark Michaelson, Mike Smith, Theresa Dougherty, Ruth Davis Konigsberg, and the team at *Men's Health* Books.

The editors of *Men's Health* and *Women's Health* magazines, especially Adam Bornstein and Adam Campbell, for their exercise expertise; Clint Carter, for his nutrition insights; Bill Phillips and Steve Borkowski for their Web and marketing support; and Lisa Bain and Peter Moore, for their inspiring calm and professionalism.

The staff of *Best Life* magazine, especially Heather Hurlock, whose contribution to this book was invaluable.

Karen Rinaldi, Chris Krogermeier, Beth Lamb, Erin Williams, and the team at Rodale Books.

Fotoulla Euripidou, Meridith Lampert, and Philavong Chanda for their dedication to getting just the facts, ma'am. Allison Falkenberry, Agnes Hansdorfer, Brett LeVecchio, Erin Clinton, and Allison Keane, who have helped us to spread the word about the *Women's Health* Diet.

Elaine Kaufman, for her heaping plates of wisdom and encouragement.

And my daughters Dominique, Anaïs, and Zoë, without whom I would have a lot more money—and a lot less joy.

INTRODUCTION
WIN THE WAR ON FAT

It's time to gain control of your weight with the *Women's Health* Secrets of the Slim.

Inside your body, at this very moment, there's a war going on: a battle between the cells that make up muscle and those that make up fat.

On one side (the good side) is Muscle. Think of Muscle as your closest BFF, one who loans you her most flattering going-out top because she knows that the better you look, the more you both outshine all the other girls and the more you both get noticed.

Contrary to what you might think, Muscle does not want to make you look big and bulky. That's what Fat does. Fat is like that passive-aggressive frenemy who always says no even when those pants do make your butt look big. Muscle on the other hand keeps your belly flat, your backside firm, and your body burning calories.

Fat hates Muscle, and the feeling is mutual. Fat wants to get rid of Muscle so it can make room for more of its muffin-top-making, energy-sucking friends inside your body. Muscle wants to do away with Fat so it can torch all incoming calories and keep you looking slim and fab.

You know which side you're rooting for. But here's the problem: In this war, Fat will always have an unfair advantage. The only way Muscle can win is with your help.

The Women's Health Diet will show you how to win that battle. It will help you build muscle and burn away fat while eating the very best food on the planet and never, ever feeling hungry. It will make you stronger, sexier, leaner, and healthier than you've ever been before. And it will start to take effect, well, pretty much from your very first bite.

Ready to dig in?

A Better You, Fast

When you first picked up this book and took a glance at the flawless body of that woman on the cover, your first thought might have been, "This is going to be really hard." She seems too freakin' perfect, doesn't she, with that impossibly flat midsection? Being like that chick is totally out of reach, right?

HOT TIPS

10 TIPS THAT CAN CHANGE YOUR LIFE IN 10 SECONDS OR LESS

1 Drink Your Milk. Think you're getting a nutritional boost from your morning cereal? Up to 40 percent of the vitamins in fortified cereals dissolve in the milk. If you don't drink the leftover cow juice, you're not getting the fancy-pants nutrients!

2 Ice It, Ace It. Drink a few glasses of ice-cold water before and during exercise. Studies show that the cold stuff can improve endurance by about 23 percent. And ice water forces your body to expend calories warming it up, boosting your metabolism as well.

3 Lift, Damn It!. Verbally expressing emotion while lifting increases muscle strength by up to 25 percent. (Of course, it also increases your risk of being tossed out of the gym by the same percentage . . .) Or get someone to scream at you: You'll be able to lift 5 to 8 percent more weight if you get verbal encouragement from a trainer or workout partner.

4 Bribe Yourself Fit. Bet a colleague (like the one who's not so secretly gunning for your job) 50 bucks that you can stick to your workout program for 6 months. Studies show that those who do achieve an average 97 percent success rate. Alternate plan? Schedule your workouts, then put $5 in a jar for each one you make. Pledge the money toward something sweet, like a new bike or a trip to Vegas.

5 Pick The Red One. Red cabbage has 15 times as much wrinkle-fighting beta-carotene as green cabbage. Red bell peppers have up to nine times as much vitamin C as green ones.

6 Spear A Hangover. To reduce the severity of a hangover, order a side of asparagus. When South Korean researchers exposed a group of human liver cells to asparagus extract, the extract suppressed free radicals and more than doubled the effects of two enzymes responsible for metabolizing alcohol.

7 Listen To Your Feet. If you can hear yourself running, you're setting yourself up for injury. Pounding the pavement comes from bad form. Keep your feet close to the ground and use a quick, shuffling stride.

8 Don't Buy Wheat Bread. Huh? Isn't it good for me? Actually, "wheat bread" is often just white bread dyed with molasses to make it look dark. Look instead for "100 percent whole wheat" or "whole grain." Even better: rye bread. Swedish researchers found that 8 hours after people ate rye, they felt less hungry than those who noshed wheat bread, thanks to rye's high fiber content.

9 Cheat With A Dumbbell. Lift a dumbbell weight as many times as you can. Then, when you can't complete one more repetition, use your free hand to help push your weighted hand through another rep. Once you're at the top of the move, remove your free hand and slowly lower the weight. Studies show that negative resistance exercises like this are more effective at muscle building than standard exercises.

10 Dry Off Head To Toe. After a shower, you'll prevent a chill by drying your head and neck first. You'll also reduce the risk of anything nasty from the shower floor making its way up your body.

Wrong. *The Women's Health Diet* is a complete nutrition and fitness plan designed to transform your body quickly and easily—or, more accurately, to help your body transform itself. (Hey, why should you do all the work?) It's a complete mind-body plan that will take you exactly where you want to go: to the very best point in your life. The point at which you are the healthiest, fittest, and happiest you've ever been. And it's designed to keep you there, for decades to come.

> **HOT TIP #11**
>
> **Steel yourself.** Steel-cut oats trigger twice as many immunity-boosting white blood cells as rolled, quick-cooking oats. Sure, they take up more time, but so do sick days.

See, there are two types of women in the world. Type one: women who are on top of it all. Their hair is never weeks overdue for a trim, their outfits are always on trend, their cars are off-the-lot spotless, and a gift for their hubby's or boyfriend's next birthday—which is still 2 weeks away—is already wrapped and hidden under a sweater on the shelf of their meticulously organized closets. Women like that have no trouble keeping fit, because their refrigerators are as well-thought-out as their wardrobes and their workouts are programmed into their calendars, snuggled up right between their book groups and their Big Sister outings.

These ladies tend to show up in the expected places: the Olympics, the society pages, the Hamptons, or as the newest guest star on *Glee*.

But these women are the exceptions. Most of us won't be appearing alongside Dara Torres, Ivanka Trump, Serena Williams, or Lea Michele anytime soon. We don't have personal trainers, executive chefs, or multimillion-dollar endorsement deals. Most of us are just, well, regular mortals: We work hard, we like our downtime, and we're pretty damn good at what we do. But we're also balancing about a million and one daily dramas, demands, and drudgeries, trying to figure out the right path forward as we're bombarded on all sides by health and nutrition choices that are as twisted and tangled as a *Twilight* plot.

Any regular woman who wants to be better than she is right now, physically and mentally, needs a leg up—a little advice she can trust, a big sister who's been around the block and can help her navigate the Sudoku puzzle of life.

That's why we've created *The Women's Health Diet*. For nearly a decade, women who want to improve their bodies and their lives have been turning to *Women's Health* as the ultimate source for fitness, nutrition, and weight-loss information anywhere in the world. From its very first issue to its rapid growth into a major player with 10 international editions and 8 million readers worldwide, *Women's Health* has collected, analyzed, studied, and refined the most authoritative research ever conducted on sculpting and enhancing the female body into its fittest, healthiest form. And every bit of advice we proffer is vetted—by the latest science, by the top experts, and by our own independent testing—to ensure that it works.

At the Energy Center—our on-site fitness facility—we try out the latest exercise gear, techniques, and strategies. In our library—the largest private medical library in the world—we keep a database

> **HOT TIP #12**
>
> **Don't skip out.** There is a 61 percent likelihood that after missing one workout you'll also skip an exercise session the following week, according to a UK study. Keep that in mind the next time you consider forgoing a trip to the gym.

that tracks and sorts every study published in every top scientific journal in the world. At the Rodale Institute—the 333-acre experimental farm operated by our parent company, Rodale Inc.—we unearth the healthiest foods on the planet and discover the best ways to raise, harvest, and consume them. And in our test kitchens and company cafeterias, we even cook up and taste test those foods, using recipes we've honed through years of nutritional research.

Along the way, we've discovered that fitness and nutrition are at the core of just about every area a woman can hope to improve on in her life, from looking great to gaining solid financial footing (one study at New York University found that people who carry an extra 40 pounds make 20 percent less than their slimmer colleagues) to improving her whole outlook on life (nutrients in the *Women's Health* Diet, like folate and omega-3 fatty acids, have been shown to boost intelligence, mood, and even sexual health). And we've tapped every expert source of information for every conundrum facing the modern woman, from how to nix shaving bumps (dissolve two aspirin in 3 tablespoons of facial toner and apply to the affected area) to how to get a better abs workout (you can do 17 percent more situps if you're properly hydrated, studies show) to how to trick yourself into eating less (scientists at the University of Massachusetts found that people who turn off the TV before eating consume an average of 288 fewer calories). It's that kind of authoritative research that has gone into designing the Secrets of the Slim, the backbone of the Women's Health Diet, and informs the tips sprinkled throughout these pages.

And that's why you can trust us when we say that the distance between where you are now and where you want to be is smaller than you think.

HOT TIP #13

A roll in the hay keeps the doctor away. People who have sex once or twice a week have stronger immune systems than people who have sex less than once a week, according to a study at Wilkes University.

An Extraordinary Plan for Ordinary Women

Think about this: With each passing decade of her life, a woman's ability to burn calories slows by about 5 percent. While it may seem like you're destined to expand like bread dough as you get older, reversing that course doesn't require as dramatic of a life change as you might think. When USDA scientists studied the eating habits of 8,837 adults, they found that on a typical day, overweight adults eat a mere 100 calories more than their normal-weight peers—the equivalent of having a cookie with your 3 p.m. coffee.

A hundred calories? Come on! Really? If that's true, then why does it seem so hard for most of us to get the bodies we want? Why do we feel miles away from the Albas, Biels, and Anistons of the world?

Because we're surrounded by a world of bad: bad advice, bad choices, and above all, bad food. (That includes plenty of stuff being marketed as "health food.") The fact is, trusting food manufacturers to watch over your body is like trusting Amy Winehouse to pick up your prescriptions. Thanks to our nutritionally bankrupt food supply, two out of every three of the girls you went to high school with are now overweight or obese. (If they weren't already that way when you were sitting next to them in algebra class. The percentage of kids ages 12 to 19 who qualify as obese nearly quadrupled between the mid-1970s and the mid-2000s.) How did this happen?

It wasn't some tsunami of fat that washed over us all. It was just 100 calories a day. Today and yesterday and the day before that...

Well, guess what? Tomorrow is a brand-new day.

> **HOT TIP #14**
>
> **Go dark.**
> In almost every case, the darker the color of a bean or vegetable, the more nutrients it contains. Black beans beat navy beans and broccoli tops cauliflower, every time.

Rebuilding a Better You

If you've tried diet and fitness plans before, you've probably discovered one serious problem with most of them: They're about sacrificing, about cutting down, about giving up.

Who likes that?

But the *Women's Health* Diet is different, in several ways:

IT'S ABOUT LIVING YOUR BEST LIFE. One of the coolest aspects of the *Women's Health* Diet is that you can pretty much cheat anytime you want—as long as you're cheating with the best. Ice cream? Sure. Nachos? Okay. Gooey delivery pizza? Yes, actually. You can indulge your taste buds any time you want, but with one small caveat: You're only allowed to indulge in THE BEST. That means the best-tasting, healthiest, smartest versions of your favorite foods—even foods that come at you through your car window. (The *Women's Health* 250 Best Foods for Women can be found in Chapter 10.) Once you discover that you can still order a burger from the drive-through, but save 800 flab-inducing calories and increase your muscle-building protein intake simply by choosing the best of the best, you'll see how very easy this diet plan is!

IT'S ABOUT WORKING WITH YOUR BODY, NOT AGAINST IT. The groundbreaking science that's emerged in just the past year has shown that when it comes to food, timing is everything. In fact, your body goes through periods every day when it wants to burn fat, build muscle, and grow leaner and stronger—it just needs the right fuel at the right time. (That's why we'll have you eating

> **HOT TIP #15**
>
> **Cut the paper.**
> In a Cornell study, people who ate from paper plates with plastic utensils tended to consider their food just a snack, while those who ate the same food off "real" plates considered their food a meal. Result: Those who eat off paper plates are more likely to seek out food later.

the majority of your calories in the first half of the day.) Simply by knowing how to time your meals, you'll prime your body for maximum muscle and superfast weight loss—and you'll stave off hunger pangs.

IT'S ABOUT EATING MORE, NOT LESS. More good food, the kind of stuff your body craves. In fact, eating as much food as your body needs will actually be a challenge: Food is the fuel that will burn away fat and build lean, strong muscle. That's the philosophy behind what we call the *Women's Health* Nutrition System, built around eight superfoods that will help you get lean, fast. (In fact, you'll know them by the acronym FAST & LEAN, as you'll learn in the coming pages.) You'll be eating up to six times a day—three meals, a couple of snacks, even dessert. (Like we said, it's a lot of food!)

> **HOT TIP #16**
>
> **Bone up.** Research suggests that omega-3s in salmon can boost bone density. Next time you barbecue, switch beef burgers for salmon patties.

IT'S ABOUT GROWING STRONGER. Too many diets are about downsizing your body by any means possible. But the *Women's Health* Diet is about upgrading. You'll learn more about that war that's raging inside your body, the war between fat and muscle. Who wins that war will determine not just what your body will look like, but also how well, and how long, it will continue to function. (Get ready to put on your butt-kicking shoes!)

IT'S ABOUT HAVING FUN. The *Women's Health* Fast-Track Tone-Up Plan (see Chapter 8) is an incredibly efficient fitness plan that begins with three 30-minute strength training sessions per week. It's not based on sweat and sacrifice, but instead requires you to enjoy yourself. Sure, there's some work involved, but once you understand the physiological principles of stress management and active rest—whether that means walking your dog, in-line skating in the park, hitting the slopes, or jumping in the surf—you'll see just how critical having fun is to reaching your fitness goals.

Get Ready to Change Your Life!

As editors of *Women's Health* magazine, and as part of the *Men's Health* brand, we're lucky to be part of one of the greatest health and fitness teams ever assembled. But we're also something else: We're living examples of the advice we dish out every month.

You'd think it would be a no-brainer for us. After all, we get to review all the latest diet studies, meet with the most sought-after nutrition experts, try the newest fitness equipment, and taste-test the healthiest foods. (Yeah, we're not complaining.) It's easy to imagine that we hold meetings while snacking on kale chips, sipping cucumber juice, and performing sun salutations. And that all these healthy habits mean we march boldly into our high school reunions bursting with confidence and that all the clothes in our wardrobe are the same size and fit us perfectly.

Sigh. We wish!

The fact is, there's not one editor on staff who hasn't struggled with her (or his!) body in some way. From a nagging self-consciousness about a flabby butt to post-pregnancy pounds that refuse to budge, we have personally experienced it all.

But a funny thing happens to people when they come to work at *Women's Health*: They start following the kind of fitness, nutrition, and stress-management advice we publish in every issue. Like the woman who didn't move a muscle for 4 years after having a baby but can now check a triathlon off her bucket list—and see her abs

---

HOT TIP #17

Shut up and eat. The louder your surroundings, the less sweet or salty food tastes (and the more crunchy it seems). You're more likely to add more of the bad stuff if you're surrounded by chaos. Bad news for any sad creature who has ever been lured into Chuck E. Cheese's.

for the first time in her life. Or the editor who traded artificial "diet" foods for natural and organic ones—and has through-the-roof energy and glowing skin to show for it. Or the one who asked for a raise because living the *Women's Health* way caused all of her clothes to suddenly become too big in the waist (too bad we don't get clothing allowances around here!) .

The kind of thinking that goes into producing *Women's Health* has literally changed our lives for the better. And it's changed the lives of millions of other women as well. Now, it's your turn.

Look, we know that most diets aren't fun. Burning calories while eating fewer of them has a way of making you pretty darn miserable. But the *Women's Health* Diet approaches weight loss in an entirely different way than most other plans out there. Instead of depriving yourself of food, *you'll actually eat more and won't feel hungry*! Instead of logging long hours of soul-crushing cardio, *you'll learn how to burn fat efficiently—and spend less time exercising*! And instead of losing weight just to gain it all back once the "diet" is over, *you'll set in motion permanent lifestyle changes that will make staying on track easier than ever.*

The end result? A leaner, healthier, more confident you.

Let the *Women's Health* Diet change your life. You'll be glad you did.

JUMPSTART
A QUICK LOOK AT THE PRINCIPLES OF THE
WOMEN'S HEALTH DIET

HOW TO GET FAST & LEAN:
THE *WOMEN'S HEALTH* NUTRITION SYSTEM

WHAT TO EAT The *Women's Health* Diet is based on eight superfood groups, foods scientifically proven to get you lean, fast. In fact, all you need to remember is:

Fiber-rich grains
Avocados, oils, and healthy fats
Spinach and leafy greens
Turkey and lean meats

Legumes
Eggs and dairy
Apples and other fruits
Nuts and seeds

+ Quality protein, mood-boosting folate, brain-building omega-3s, and fiber-rich carbs like whole fruits and vegetables

— Refined carbs, salt, high-fructose corn syrup and other sweeteners, and trans fats

HOW MUCH TO EAT Instead of counting calories or obsessing over portion sizes, pack your plate with nutrient-dense, fiber-rich foods; pay attention to your body's signals; and eat only until you're full. General portion guidelines can be found in the palm of your hand. Literally, as in:

MEATS: The size of your palm
VEGETABLES AND FRUITS:
The size of a tight fist
OILS AND OTHER HEALTHY
FATS: A teaspoon is equal to the end

of your thumb, from the knuckle up
LEGUMES: Whatever fits in the palm
of your hand
GRAINS: The size of a tight fist
DAIRY: The size of your palm

5 MEALS	CALORIES PER MEAL		+ BEVERAGES/DESSERT 100 to 200		
	BREAKFAST	**SNACK**	**LUNCH**	**SNACK**	**DINNER**
	500 to 600	150 to 200	300 to 400	150 to 200	300 to 400

The *Women's Health* Diet is about eating more food, not less. By following our Secrets of the Slim, you will fill up on the nutrients you need to stoke your metabolism, blast belly fat, and build lean, long-lasting muscle. Here's a quick overview of what you'll be eating each day:

THE *WOMEN'S HEALTH* FAST-TRACK TONE-UP PLAN

The *Women's Health* Fast-Track Tone-Up Plan will turbocharge your weight loss. It is a revolutionary new workout based around time—not around boring sets. You'll move quickly from one exercise to the next, doing as many reps as you can in 30 seconds, then resting for 15 seconds before moving on to the next exercise.

WEIGHT WORKOUTS PER WEEK **3**

DURATION OF WORKOUTS IN MINUTES 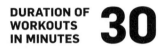 **30**

ADDITIONAL FAT-BURNING ACTIVITIES: Choose from a wide variety of fun activities, from hiking to tennis to playing tag with your kids. A weekly session of "having fun" is a mandatory part of your new workout plan!

THE *WOMEN'S HEALTH* SECRETS OF THE SLIM

SLIM SECRET #1: "I Will Eat Protein with Every Meal and Every Snack." (Eat 10–15 grams per snack, 30 per meal.)

SLIM SECRET #2: "I Will Never Eat the World's Worst Breakfast." (The worst breakfast is no breakfast at all.)

SLIM SECRET #3: "I Will Eat Before and After Exercise." (Eat a mix of protein and carbs.)

SLIM SECRET #4: "I Will Eat It if It Grows on a Tree." (Add as many fruits, vegetables, nuts, and beans to your diet as you can stomach.)

SLIM SECRET #5: "I Will Become a Salad Savant." (Eat them before your meals, not in place of them!)

SLIM SECRET #6: "I Will Not Drink Sugar Water." (Watch your beverage calories.)

SLIM SECRET #7: "I Will Follow the Secrets ~~100 Percent~~ 80 Percent of the Time." (The *Women's Health* Diet lets you cheat whenever you want!)

1

LEANER.
STRONGER.
SEXIER.
Make all three of those words describe you with the help of *The Women's Health Diet.*

It's time to transform your body. If you're like a lot of women, you may feel like you are constantly struggling with your weight. Or perhaps you find yourself stuck in a baby-carrots-and-cardio rut that's just not working anymore. Whatever your motivation, the Women's Health Diet is here to help you make your goal of a healthier, more attractive body a reality.

The first and easiest step to achieving the body you've always wanted is changing the way you think about food. As Megan Tretter, who lost 28 pounds on the *Women's Health* Diet in just 6 weeks and toned up her entire body, explained, "I wouldn't call it a diet but more of an attitude change. Instead of seeing food as either guilty pleasure or penance, I now look at it as fuel," she said.

Something is clearly wrong with the way we approach eating. According to a 2010 study in the *Journal of the American Medical Association*, although our nation's obesity rates may finally have stopped rising, that still leaves a whopping 64 percent of American women either overweight or obese (defined as a BMI of 25 or higher).

Our obesity epidemic has become a massive threat to public health. According to the National Institutes of Health, the health care costs associated with obesity are expected to double every decade. And it's not solely an American problem: According to some estimates, by the year 2030, nearly 2 billion people around the globe will be overweight or obese.

Now, we know what you may be thinking: "So all I need to do is lay off the Snickers bars and start running more, right?" Not quite. Because while you probably know some heavy folks who have brought extra weight on themselves, surely you also know people who watch what they eat, try to exercise regularly, even put themselves on strict diet plans, and still pack on the pounds—losing a few inches here and there only to wind up bigger than ever. And evidence is mounting that our weight isn't solely our fault. Something else is at work.

> **HOT TIP #18**
>
> **Push away fat.**
> The pushup is a good indicator of whether you're exercising enough now to avoid fat later, according to a Canadian study. The researchers found that people who perform poorly in a pushup test are 78 percent more likely to gain 20 pounds of flab over the next two decades.

She lost 15 pounds in 6 weeks!

SUCCESS stories

"Wow, this is incredible!"

MARLYN STEWART, 33, Houston, Texas

STARTING WEIGHT 175 LB / WEIGHT AFTER 6 WEEKS 160 LB / HEIGHT 5'4"

Weight Watchers, Jenny Craig, Atkins, you name it. Marlyn Stewart has tried them all. But her scale never budged, at least not permanently. Desperate, she tried the *Women's Health* Diet. "It changed my life," Marlyn said.

A Total-Body Transformation

Marlyn was ready for a change, so she prepared herself to get disciplined. "I'd leave myself little reminders to stick to it." But staying on track wasn't a problem. "There was always something new—new recipes, new workouts—so I never got bored." And when the weight started melting away, she was overjoyed. "Just looking at the changes in my body, I thought, 'Wow, this is incredible!'"

And she felt better, too. "I used to feel bloated all the time. Now I'm not as flabby and I have flatter abs," she said. Some other perks? Marlyn's hair got shinier, her nails grew, even her acne cleared up. Now she has fewer PMS symptoms and tons more energy. "I'm not as stressed and I'm no longer craving chocolate!"

Getting Personal

"All my friends noticed that I was happier and more fit," Marlyn said. "They wanted to know what was making me feel so good. They thought I was on medication!" So she gave them a copy of the plan, and they began to see results as well. "One friend lost almost 20 pounds and has never looked better." Even Marlyn's mom jumped on the bandwagon and wound up losing nearly 15 pounds, along with her chronic psoriasis.

In the end, the *Women's Health* Diet made Marlyn feel like someone was supporting her, and that kept her motivated. She especially liked the combination of the meal plans and guidelines. "The food was put together in ways that I wouldn't have thought of myself," she said.

The "something else" is the starve-yourself-thin, spend-your-life-in-the-gym ethos that we've been told we need to adopt in order to lose weight. Weight-loss gurus will tell you it's all a matter of willpower, but that's just not the truth. In fact, most plans are designed for short-term success but long-term failure. The *Women's Health* Diet has been created to change this picture and to help you transform your body into what it should be—a fat-burning machine. In just 6 weeks, you could lose up to 15 pounds—or more!—while toning every inch and sculpting your dream body. To initiate this change, you won't need to drastically overhaul your life, either. That's because the *Women's Health* Diet has been crafted with you in mind—your body, your schedule, your time.

> **HOT TIP #19**
>
> **Check your ego at the door.** Researchers at the University of Texas found that those who took up exercise mainly to improve appearance experienced a drop in feelings of self-worth. If you want to remind yourself why it's important to stay fit, try hanging a family photo on your exercise-room wall.

The main components of the plan are seven simple-to-follow rules—we call them the Secrets of the Slim. They're seven easy steps you'll take that will keep you making the right food choices for your body, without having to make serious sacrifices. (Slim Secret #2: "I will never eat the world's worst breakfast." That's all you need to do to start reshaping your body!) When you follow the Secrets of the Slim, weight loss isn't just easy—it's automatic!

Plus, you'll build your meals around the *Women's Health* Nutrition System—a group of eight superhealthy superfoods that will fuel weight loss, build your energy and even boost your mood. (You'll know these foods by the simple acronym FAST & LEAN—learn more about them in Chapter 7!) And just to make things even easier, we've included recipes for terrific new fat-burning foods,

Megan lost 28 pounds in 6 weeks!

SUCCESS *stories*

"This really makes me happy!"

MEGAN TRETTER, 40, Missoula, Montana

STARTING WEIGHT 280 LB / **WEIGHT AFTER 6 WEEKS 252 LB** / **HEIGHT 6'**

Megan Tretter was looking for a change from a litany of failed diets. Already an avid reader of *Women's Health*, she decided to try the *Women's Health* Diet because she knew that the information was coming from a trusted source. What she didn't realize was how the plan contained so many evidence-based strategies culled from our wealth of knowledge and experience.

Taking the First Step

Megan had found other diet programs to be too expensive and too hard to follow throughout the entire day. She was initially worried about fitting new eating habits into her schedule but soon discovered that the eating plan was not only easy to stick to, it was her favorite part.

"I really enjoyed the food part of it," she said. "I wouldn't call it a diet but more of a food attitude change. Instead of seeing food as guilty pleasure or penance, "I now view food as fuel. It actually makes meals a lot less stressful." Tips such as drinking milk in the morning before breakfast and eating before and after workouts primed her body and eliminated hunger pangs.

Feeding a Healthy Family

Megan got her husband and two kids to share in her new healthy eating habits. And as a result, they've all gotten a boost in energy that has allowed them to be more active as a family. "My daughters love it," she said. "This really makes me happy."

Reaching New Milestones

As the pounds came off, Megan discovered that her body had new capabilities. Although she calls herself a beginner, she says she's "lost enough weight to begin running." It was that accomplishment that inspired her current fitness goal—to run a half marathon.

and a list of the 250 Best Foods for Women. Sample any of them at any time, and watch the pounds disappear!

Now, more and more women are discovering that the Women's Health Diet really works. Consider the story of one of our testers, Marlyn Stewart. By age 33, she'd packed 175 pounds onto her 5'4" frame and had tried diet after diet to get rid of those unwanted pounds—never with much success. But then she discovered the *Women's Health* Diet, and everything changed.

> **HOT TIP #20**
>
> **Romp rigorously.**
> One vigorous go-around in the bedroom blasts about 200 calories and doubles your heart rate. Twice a week? Shed nearly 6 pounds a year.

None of the many diets that Marlyn had tried had kept her motivated. She'd lose some weight only to have it come right back when she fell off the wagon. But with the meal plans, guidelines, and food suggestions in the *Women's Health* Diet, she always felt like someone had her back. "It felt like someone was personally guiding me," she said. What's more, not only did Marlyn lose weight on the program and feel less bloated, her body responded in other surprising ways. "My hair, skin, and nails improved, and my abs got flatter!"

By combining new healthy eating habits with regular workouts, she saw her body become fitter and sexier. And Marlyn also enjoyed another huge benefit: Once plagued by PMS mood swings, she felt her symptoms dramatically diminish. "I had more energy and felt less stressed and happier overall," she said. Her friends all noticed the transformation, too. "They wanted to know what I was doing that made me look and feel so good!"

Is it possible that one plan can help you create total mind and body change? Absolutely. And what incredible effects you'll see. Here's just a short list of the many ways the *Women's Health* Diet will change your life:

You'll Eat More Than Ever—and Never Feel Hungry!

Here's a fact about most diets: They're setting you up for failure. If you've ever tried a restrictive diet program before, you know what we're talking about. These plans are focused on "good" foods and "bad" foods, extensive calorie-counting or cutting entire food groups out of your life. But you can only deprive your body of something for so long; sooner or later, denying that craving for a slice of cheese pizza could lead you to the moment when you break down and eat half the pie, or more. The good news is, there is no restriction on the *Women's Health* Diet.

Instead, throughout the day you'll spread your eating over five meals and snacks created from eight superfood groups, each designed to get you on the fast track to lean. In fact, that's what we've called these foods: FAST & LEAN. You'll read all about them in Chapter 7. With the right combination of whole foods, all chock-full of belly-filling fiber, protein, and other key nutrients, you'll end up eating more food but fewer calories, which is the perfect formula for weight-loss success.

And it's a formula that's been proven time and again: A 2007 study in the *American Journal of Clinical Nutrition* compared the weight loss of two groups: One group was instructed to eat a lot of whole foods (like those in the *Women's Health* Diet FAST & LEAN plan), while the other group was instructed to eat a low-fat diet. The whole-foods group ate 25 percent more food by volume and still lost an average of 5 pounds more weight. How? They were eating fewer calories, but they were still satisfied, thanks to the foods' high nutrient and water content.

And that's what happens when you follow the *Women's Health* Diet, because you replace junk calories with nutrition calories.

Indeed, a study in the *Journal of Food Composition and Analysis* determined that nearly one-third of the food most people eat is pure junk. Five food groups—sweets and desserts, soft drinks, fruit drinks, salty snacks, and alcohol—make up 30 percent of our calories. (Soda alone contributes more than 7 percent of the average person's daily calories!)

HOT TIP #21

Think before you eat. British researchers found that people who reviewed their previous meals before chowing down ate 30 percent fewer calories than those who didn't. The theory: simply remembering what you've already eaten makes you less likely to overindulge.

So your best weight-loss bet is not to eat less food; it's to eat more. But it needs to be food that's high in nutrition and low in empty calories and fat-promoting ingredients. And on the *Women's Health* Diet that's easy to accomplish. You fuel your body with the finest foods out there. And when you need a break from the FAST & LEAN superfoods? Cheat at will, but do it with the very best cheat foods in the world, from fast-food burgers to delivery pizza. And we've done most of the hard work for you. With our list of the 250 Best Foods for Women (you'll find it in Chapter 10), you can customize this plan to fit your tastes, your goals—your life!

You'll Lose Fat—and Sculpt a Sexy Body!

Too many diet plans restrict calories, which is a really great way to lose weight in the short run—and gain it all back, and more, in the long run.

You've heard the term "yo-yo dieting" before, but you probably don't know what triggers the yo-yo effect. Blame it on evolution: When your ancient ancestors had trouble finding food—because of

She lost 15 pounds!

SUCCESS *stories*

"I lost inches everywhere!"

VICKIE B., 48, Nashville, Tennessee

STARTING WEIGHT **195 LB** / WEIGHT AFTER 6 WEEKS **180 LB** / HEIGHT **5'3"**

Vickie B. was looking for a healthy way to lose weight. And once she began the program, she not only shed pounds, she also found a stress-free eating strategy that she could use for life.

Finding the Right Plan

Vickie had tried diets before but without success—one low-carb plan left her with insane cravings. The *Women's Health* Diet was a lifestyle change she could live with.

"I have to be in the office early, so eating a lot early worked for me, and I had time for the workouts at night," she said. Because the diet plan fit so easily into her schedule, it helped eliminate many problems. "I didn't get that nauseated hungry feeling [from not eating frequently enough] and then grab whatever was handy." She had more energy throughout the day, no longer experienced the "crash" that comes after empty calories, and generally felt better overall.

Replacing Fat with Muscle

On the *Women's Health* Diet, Vickie saw a dramatic change in her body. She went from a size 16 to a size 12 in just 6 weeks! And once she added the *Women's Health* Fast-Track Tone-Up Plan to her schedule, she had less back pain, and both her strength and stamina increased. She even decided to train for a half marathon.

"I have lost weight, but more important, I have lost inches everywhere," she said.

Loving the Results

Vickie said that it was seeing the pounds and inches come off that kept her motivated on the diet. But she wasn't the only person who noticed—her family and friends also commented on the changes.

"I really love my body again; I look toned and healthy," she said. "I want to lose even more and be really healthy!"

a prolonged drought, an ice age, or maybe a shortage of bows and arrows at the Neanderthal Cabela's—their bodies needed to be able to weather the hard times by using stored body mass to keep vital organs functioning. And guess what kind of tissue a hungry body burns first?

Muscle.

Here's why: Muscle burns a lot of calories—about 6 calories a day per pound. Fat, on the other hand, burns a mere 2 calories a day. So if your body is in starvation mode and needs to conserve calories, what weight will it want to drop? Right—the stuff that's using the most available calories: muscle weight. (Meanwhile, it will do everything it can to hold on to the calorically undemanding flab.) Sure, when you restrict calories, you lose fat, but you lose muscle too. And with it, you lose muscle's fat-burning power. A study in the *Journal of Applied Physiology* found that calorie restriction (decreasing caloric intake by 16 to 20 percent) decreases bone mass, muscle mass, and strength.

> **HOT TIP #22**
>
> **Don't crowd your chow.** When picking food from a buffet, leave spaces between the foods you select. You could consume up to 20 percent fewer calories than if you pack your plate.

And that's exactly what happens when we follow a traditional diet. Once we stop "dieting," we go back to the same way of eating—but this time, without that valuable calorie burn we got from having more muscle. The more restrictive the diet, the more muscle you lose, the more flab you'll gain over the long haul.

But the *Women's Health* Diet doesn't require you to starve yourself, cut out your favorite foods, or lose muscle. And if you incorporate the *Women's Health* Fast-Track Tone-Up Plan into your weight-loss program, you'll actually build muscle and burn even more calories!

She toned her entire body in 6 weeks!

"I feel sharper and more alert!"

BETH KANE, 30, Austin, Texas

STARTING WEIGHT **148 LB** / WEIGHT AFTER 6 WEEKS **143 LB** / HEIGHT **5'10"**

Beth Kane had been dieting on and off since the age of 14, but could never stick to a plan . . . until she found the *Women's Health* Diet.

Seeing—and Feeling—a Difference

Beth's initial goal wasn't to lose weight. Instead, it was to feel her best in her body and look amazing, day in and day out. "I'm always game to lose a pound or two, but this time it was more about feeling stronger, better, and firmer as opposed to losing digits on the scale," she said.

Not only did she lose pounds and notice that her clothes fit better, she toned her entire body as well. She saw more definition in her arms and legs, and both her husband and friends commented on her newly slimmer physique. "The *Women's Health* Fast-Track Tone-Up Plan helped me see the results more quickly than if I had just tried the diet alone," Beth said.

Feeling Mentally Stronger, Too

Beth's body went through more than just a physical transformation. "About 2 weeks in, I started to feel sharper and more alert," she said. "I credit that to eating a more balanced diet throughout the day at logical intervals." No stranger to other diet options, she was particularly impressed with the results of two of the plan's guidelines: eating breakfast and including protein with each meal. "On days I didn't follow that advice, I felt sluggish and continually hungry."

And feeling good is what keeps Beth on the *Women's Health* Diet. "I want to look good," she said, "but most of all, I want to feel fit. I don't want to struggle climbing the stairs. Or feel my stomach fat vibrate when I'm driving down the road. And the *Women's Health* Diet has helped me feel and look better. I'm a huge, huge fan!"

You'll Have More Energy and See Fast Results!

Recent research suggests that when it comes to eating—and, ultimately, shedding fat and building muscle—*when* you eat is just as important as *what* you eat. On the *Women's Health* Diet, you'll be providing your body with the fuel it needs when it needs it the most—in the morning and before and after you work out.

According to one study, your risk of obesity increases 450 percent if you regularly skip breakfast. That's right—450 percent. But by consuming a protein-rich morning meal, you'll pull your body out of the fuel-deprived state it was in while you were sleeping and into the fat-burning, muscle-promoting zone. A 2008 study at Virginia Commonwealth University found that people who ate a large, protein-rich breakfast lost significantly more weight than those who consumed smaller morning meals with less protein. Unfortunately, our food industry has conditioned us into scarfing refined carbs in the morning, which is the exact opposite of what we need. *The Women's Health Diet* will show you how to fight back against crazy morning carbo-loading and get the protein you need to fuel your body and keep you burning fat all day and all night.

You'll also be able to build even more muscle by scheduling your meals around your workouts. Dutch and British researchers reported that eating before exercise speeds muscle growth and helps your body increase strength and burn fat more effectively. Plus, independent studies by Finnish and British sci-

HOT TIP #23

Bribe yourself slim. When a craving hits, bribe yourself thin. Instead of munching, put money into a box every time you want a snack. The growing pile of dough will be a reminder that you can overpower your urges. When you've saved enough cash, use it to splurge on a non-food reward.

entists discovered that, in addition to helping you develop lean muscle faster, eating a balance of protein and carbs both before and after exercise can speed your recovery time and help to reduce soreness after a tough workout.

You'll Protect Your Body from Disease— Without Drugs!

Folate is crucial for proper brain and body functioning, according to Harvard researchers. A study in the *American Journal of Clinical Nutrition* found that people with low folate levels have an increased risk of impaired cognitive function and dementia. And a study in the journal *Psychotherapy and Psychosomatics* shows that low folate levels are found in depressed members of the general U.S. population. (And it's not just your mind that suffers: Folate deficiency has been implicated in most of the major diseases of our time. It leads to an increased risk of obesity, stroke, heart disease, cognitive impairment, Alzheimer's, and even cancer.)

But you can reverse your risk for all these diseases and, within weeks, see a noticeable improvement in your mood and brain function, simply by following the guidelines of *The Women's Health Diet*. Studies show that adding folate-rich greens to your diet reduces fatigue, improves energy levels, and helps battle depression—something supplements can't do.

By incorporating *The Women's Health Diet* guidelines into your daily schedule, you'll also increase your intake of omega-3 fatty acids—healthy fats that can cut your risk of everything from heart

HOT TIP #24

Embrace ginger spice. Two grams of ground ginger a day can reduce soreness and help enhance new muscle growth, say researchers.

disease and stroke to arthritis and asthma. These nutrients are essential in boosting your mood and promoting brain health. Research suggests that people with a diet high in omega 3-rich foods live longer and carry less abdominal fat than those who don't. And don't worry if you're not a seafood eater: Omega-3s can be found in a multitude of other foods, from walnuts to kiwifruit.

Plus, not only are the foods you'll find in the *Women's Health* Nutrition System healthier for you, they're tastier, too. Why? Because our taste buds evolved to crave flavor, and foods get their flavors from nutrients. The tangy tartness of berries comes from their massive vitamin loads, the fat in fish delivers healthy omega-3s, and the bittersweet taste of chocolate carries a dose of antioxidants.

You'll Rev Up Your Sex Life!

A survey of 1,210 people of different weights and sizes conducted by researchers at Duke University Medical Center showed that obese people were 25 times as likely to report dissatisfaction with sex as normal weight people. To make things worse, a diet high in saturated and trans fasts actually lowers your libido by decreasing your sex hormones. The good news? The *Women's Heath* Diet reverses this equation, slims down your body and boosts your sexual pleasure. Several studies have shown that people report much greater enjoyment of sexual activity following just a 10 percent weight loss, says Martin Binks, PhD, clinical director of Binks Behavioral Health and an assistant consulting professor at Duke University Medical Center. With the *Women's Health* Diet, you'll look sexier, which means that you'll feel sexier too.

Even those of us who don't need to shed a lot of pounds will see improvements in the sack by using the *Women's Health* Fast-Track Tone-Up Plan. According to research done at the Meston Sexual Psychophysiology Laboratory at the University of Texas in Austin, exercise sparks a woman's libido by as much as 150 percent by activating your central nervous system and preparing your body for arousal. But there's another reason that exercise leads to better sex. Many of the same issues that cause erectile dysfunction in men—high blood pressure, high cholesterol—can also lead to sexual dysfunction in women. Good sex requires good cardiovascular health; impaired blood flow is not just a man's problem.

So there you have it. What's not to love about a plan that allows you to eat better versions of the foods you love, all while helping you become a stronger, healthier, happier version of you? It's time to get started! Your new body is waiting.

HOT TIP #25

Arm yourself.
Want sculpted, toned arms? Stop concentrating on your biceps. Triceps—the muscles on the back of your upper arm—make up 70 percent of your upper arm musculature. Focus on these to lose the jelly arms.

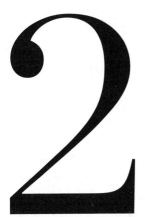

HOW FIT ARE YOU?
Take the *Women's Health* Fitness Assessment and discover your body's strengths—and its weaknesses.

Wild guess: You're pretty stoked when you can check off three 30-minute cardio sessions a week. Throw in some crunches while watching *Mad Men*, maybe a few lunges, a couple of go-to arm moves, and you're golden, right? You've got a fitness plan and you're sticking to it.

If you're like a lot of us, once you find a workout that's comfortable, there's no changing it up. But over time, a comfortable routine, especially a cardio rut, won't challenge your body enough to really transform it. In fact, it's a one-way ticket to the land of limited results, a.k.a. the dreaded "plateau."

Nor will a comfortable routine counteract the detriments of the typical daily grind: Long days slumped over in front of the computer, endless commutes wedged into the driver's seat or subway car—hours upon hours, week after week, in which your body is doing something it just wasn't built to do. Over time, as you remain locked into bad postures, some muscles get shortened and tightened, others get stretched and weakened, and the natural alignment of your body gets tweaked until it's totally out of whack. And even if you manage to work out regularly, your if-it-ain't-broke plan isn't going to fix what's coming slowly, inexorably undone.

HOT TIP #26

Keep your mouth busy. Chew gum while you prepare food or whenever you're surrounded by stuff you don't need to eat.

That's because almost everyone who hits the gym (or works out at home) commits the cardinal sin of exercise: poor form. Most people don't know how to perform the most basic exercises correctly, and that "complementary" training session you got when you signed up at the gym didn't necessarily arm you with all the tools you need to make a real difference. Poor exercise technique is the number-one reason many gym-goers struggle to make real, long-lasting changes to their bodies. You can't go from flab to fab unless you identify where you're weakest, choose the right exercises to counteract those weaknesses, and perform those exercises correctly, time after time.

That's what this book will help you do. Once you know how to identify these problem areas and improve how you move, you'll get more out of your workouts—every time you exercise. In no time, the word "plateau" will be a thing of the past.

Think about it: When you perform an exercise incorrectly or focus on one or two body parts at the expense of others, it sets your body up for a series of failures. One poor rep becomes 10. Multiply that by 3 sets performed 3 times per week, and that's 90 reps of joint-aching, imbalance-creating movements. Continue the math and it becomes easy to see why you haven't experienced success, despite your best efforts. If you're doing the exercises wrong or have hidden weakness, you'll not only see limited results, you'll get hurt. In fact, a 27-year review of gym injuries found that nearly 70 percent of them were either sprains, strains, or soft tissue injuries caused by poor form. And even if you're doing the exercises correctly, you might still be sending yourself to coach potato status. That's because many exercise programs focus on vanity results rather than healthy results. Researchers at Nova Southeastern University, in Florida, found that men who lift weights are more likely to have shoulder pain and other upper body injuries that restrict exercise than those who never lift weights. The reason: Poor training programs that overemphasize the chest and biceps (typical show-off muscles for dudes) and underemphasize the muscles that protect their shoulders. Think this just happens to guys? Wrong. Bunches of crunches may chisel your tummy, but they only scratch the surface. Crunches simply can't reach the deeper core muscles and surrounding muscle systems that support the rest of your body. Now you're on the couch with an

> **HOT TIP #27**
>
> **Uncover the flax.** Sprinkle ground flaxseed over cereal, pancakes, yogurt, and smoothies. It's an easy way to add belly-filling fiber and omega-3 fatty acids. Not a fan of flax? Try pumpkin or sunflower seeds—two more great sources of healthy fats and some fiber.

ice pack instead of in the gym rocking a racer-back.

Of course, this is no reason not to work out. The benefits of exercise far outweigh the potential for injury. But a recent survey found that 64 percent of active adults under the age of 45 suffer from joint pain caused by a misunderstanding of how to correctly lift weights.

HOT TIP #28

Mix your phytos. A recent study found people get the majority of their daily phytonutrients from the same few foods. Simple switches can boost your intake of vital phytos like lutein and beta-carotene. Try swapping kale for spinach, raspberries for strawberries, and sweet potatoes for carrots.

That means that if you work out regularly, you're probably hurting yourself or cutting yourself short, whether you want to admit it or not.

Now imagine the flip side. What if you exercised in such a way that your efforts were much more effective? How much better would you look then? That reality isn't so far-fetched when you consider that your body is no different from a machine. The more efficient you make your movements, the better you'll operate.

The first step is to hop off that treadmill and get started on a strength-training routine. And you need to make absolutely sure that you're doing each exercise correctly. Researchers at the College of New Jersey found that a change in bench press technique instantly increases the amount of weight you can lift by as much as 10 percent. That's 10 percent more fat-burning power! What's more, Norwegian scientists found that when exercises are done correctly, it cuts the incidence of muscle strains by 68 percent and boosts the number of reps you can complete by 17 percent on each set.

But none of this is possible without a formal assessment that points out which areas of your body need the most work. You can do this with the help of a good trainer, or you can assess and correct your own movements. That's why we designed this simple but comprehensive test that will have you on track to becoming fit the *Women's Health* way faster than ever. While there are literally thousands of exercise variations that you can perform, only a few basic movements serve as the foundation for every exercise. Mike Robertson, CSCS, a renowned specialist in corrective bodywork, identified the five most important movements to help you figure out what you need to improve. Not only will mastering proper form in these exercises help you achieve your goals, it will also eliminate weaknesses and imbalances that lead to aches and pains. Working the muscles you can't see—like the ones deep inside your core, hips, and shoulders—can be a difficult process. But target those areas and your whole body benefits. Your posture will improve, making you look taller and leaner than ever. You'll burn through your workout more efficiently, without feeling any twinges, and see faster and more dramatic results. And you'll set yourself up for a lifetime of looking, feeling, and living leaner, sexier, and healthier.

The tests in this chapter will establish a baseline level of your fitness. No matter how you perform, don't be discouraged. The exercises that you'll complete in the *Women's Health* Fast-Track Tone-Up Plan—detailed in Chapter 7—are designed to target all the movements and muscles in your body and improve any weaknesses you identify based on these tests. So whether you have weak abs, poor shoulder stability, or lack lower-body mobility, all the exercises in the *Women's Health* Fast-Track Tone-Up Plan will come to the rescue and have you looking and feeling better than ever. After 6 weeks, come back to this initial assessment and retest your ability. Don't be surprised when you pass each test with flying colors and your body is fitter and sexier than ever.

HOT TIP #29

Shut eye, melt fat. In one study, dieters who slept 8.5 hours a night lost more body fat. Dieters who slept 5.5 hours a night lost more muscle.

The *Women's Health* Fitness Assessment

These five simple exercises will reveal what areas of your body need strengthening. Read the exercise descriptions, perform the moves, and then look at yourself in the mirror (or have a friend watch you). Use the guide below to assess your performance and identify your weaknesses.

Squat Test

HOW TO DO IT: Stand as tall as you can with your feet spread shoulder-width apart. Lower your body as far as you can by pushing your hips back and bending your knees. Pause, then slowly push yourself back to the starting position.

FRONT VIEW

ASSESS YOUR FORM: As you lower your body toward the floor, what are your knees doing? Your hips, knees, and feet should all be in a straight line. If your knees start to cave in toward each other, you're at an increased risk for a knee injury. This can be anything from wear and tear that will leave your joints aching, to a serious ligament injury, such as a torn anterior cruciate ligament or meniscus, especially common in women.

YOUR WEAKNESS: Your hips and lateral hamstrings control the movement of your lower limbs, and they keep your knees tracking properly so you don't damage any ligaments. You can improve your form and prevent your knees from giving in by strengthening your glutes and hamstrings with exercises like the dumbell straight-leg deadlift (page 178).

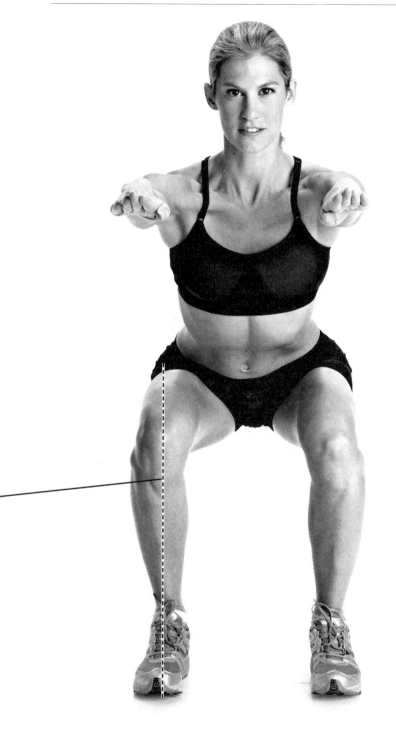

Squat Test, con't

SIDE VIEW

ASSESS YOUR FORM: As you squat, what does your chest do? It should remain upright without scrunching forward.

YOUR WEAKNESS: If your chest falls forward, it could indicate a weakness in your middle back region and can lead to neck, shoulder, or lower-back pain. Fix it by strengthening your upper back with exercises like the dumbbell row (page 187) and the pushup position dumbell row (page 179), and do foam-roller exercises along the upper portion of your back.

ASSESS YOUR FORM: As you squat down, how deep can you go without rounding your lower back? You should be able to squat until the tops of your thighs are at least parallel to the floor. And when you perform the squat with added resistance, you should be able to lower your hips below your knees, which actually protects the knees.

YOUR WEAKNESS: If you are unable to get your hips below your knees without rounding your lower back, you need to improve your hip mobility and core strength. Over time, a weak core could result in lower-back pain. Strengthen your core with exercises like cross-body mountain climbers (page 183), and loosen up your hips with foam-roller exercises like the ones at womenshealthmag.com/fitness/workout-recovery-tips.

ASSESS YOUR FORM: As you squat, where is your weight balanced? It should be toward the middle of your foot or on your heels.

YOUR WEAKNESS: If your heels come up off the floor, your quads are too strong in relation to your glutes and hamstrings. A weak backside can lead to lower-back pain or pain in the front of your knees. When you first start doing front squats in the *Women's Health* Fast-Track Tone-Up Plan, position a knee-high bench about 2 inches behind your body and squat until you sit on it. This will familiarize your body with how it feels to push your hips back. Strengthen your glutes and hamstrings with dumbbell straight-leg deadlifts (page 178).

Lunge Test

HOW TO DO IT: Stand tall with your feet hip-width apart and your hands on your hips. Step forward with your left leg and slowly lower your body until your front knee is bent at least 90 degrees. Pause, then push yourself to the starting position as quickly as you can. Repeat with your right leg.

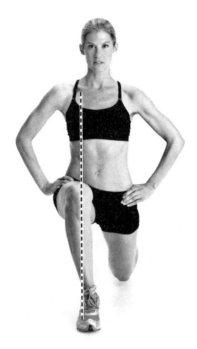

FRONT VIEW

ASSESS YOUR FORM: How do your knee and foot line up as you lower your body? When you're standing, your foot, knee, and hip should be in a straight line.

YOUR WEAKNESS: If your knee caves inward, you may have weak hip muscles. Weak hips can lead to lower-back, hip, or knee pain. Lunges work the small muscles in your hips and will offset the tightness and discomfort that results from sitting too much during the course of your day. To make the most of the exercise, do them barefoot. This improves your stability by waking up the sensory receptors on the bottom of your feet. And the more stability you have, the easier it is to create better alignment from your lower legs all the way up to your pelvis.

SIDE VIEW

ASSESS YOUR FORM: Does your torso move during the lunge? As you complete the movement, your torso should be straight up and down (perpendicular to the floor).

THE WEAKNESS: If your torso leans forward or to either side, your hip flexors may be stiff, which can lead to lower-back or knee pain. Loosen them with a hip flexor stretch like this one: Kneel on your left leg, with your right foot on the floor and right knee bent 90 degrees. Rest your hands on your hips and press your pelvis forward, feeling the stretch in your left hip flexor and quad. Hold for 30 seconds, then repeat on the right side.

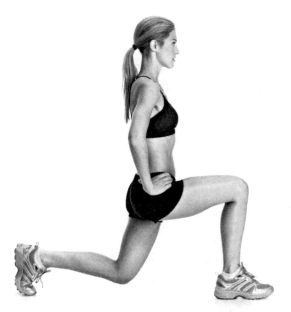

ASSESS YOUR FORM: When you do lunges, where is your weight balanced? Your body weight should be toward your midfoot or even your heel.

YOUR WEAKNESS: If your heel comes up off the floor, your quads are too strong in relation to your glutes and hamstrings. A weak backside can lead to lower-back pain or pain in the front of your knees. Whenever you lunge, watch yourself in a mirror. Think about standing tall and dropping down straight, rather than rocking forward or backward. If this doesn't work, place a knee-high bench a few inches in front of your body. This will prevent your knees from drifting forward when you lunge.

Pushup Test

HOW TO DO IT: Get down on all fours and place your hands on the floor so that they're slightly wider than shoulder-width apart. Walk your hands forward until your body forms a stright line from your shoulders to ankles. You should be at the top of a pushup position, resting your weight on your hands and your toes. Lower your body until your chest nearly touches the floor. Pause at the bottom and then push yourself back to the starting position as quickly as possible.

SIDE VIEW

ASSESS YOUR FORM: Does your torso move during the exercise? Your body should be rigid and form a straight line from your head to your ankles. Your legs should be straight, your stomach and glutes tight, and your chest open.

YOUR WEAKNESS: Too often, your lower back will sag as you transition from the lowering to the lifting phase of a pushup. This indicates weak abs or stiff hip flexors, which can lead to lower-back pain. To improve, try incline pushups as described above.

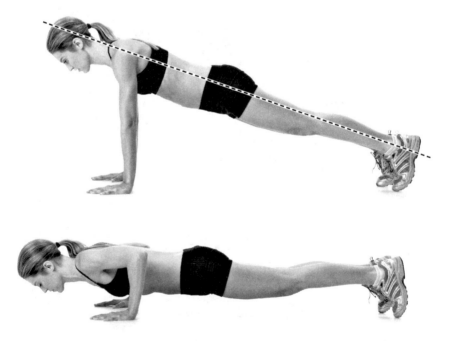

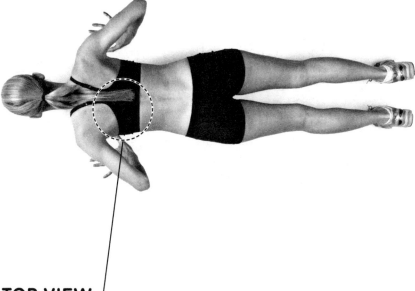

TOP VIEW

ASSESS YOUR FORM: You'll need a friend to watch you on this one. Do your shoulder blades move when you lower your body toward the floor? As you perform the pushup, your shoulder blades should stay stable and not protrude outward.

YOUR WEAKNESS: If your shoulder blades protrude outward, you have a weak serratus anterior muscle, which is located on the side of your chest along your ribs and attaches to and allows you to rotate your shoulder blade. Weakness in your serratus can lead to shoulder pain. To improve your pushup form and increase your strength, place a barbell on the pins of a squat rack at hip height and perform a pushup with your hands on the bar. As you improve, lower the bar closer to the floor until you can do a pushup on the floor with perfect form. (You can also try this on a staircase, moving to a lower step as your strength improves.)

Front Plank Test

HOW TO DO IT: Get into a pushup position but bend your elbows and rest your weight on your forearms instead of your hands. Your body should form a straight line from your shoulders to your ankles. Brace your core by contracting your abs, as if you were about to be hit in the belly. Count for how many seconds you can hold this optimal alignment. Your eventual goal should be 60 seconds.

SIDE VIEW

ASSESS YOUR FORM: Once in position, does any part of your body move? This exercise tests strength and endurance in your core and trunk muscles. Your body should be rigid and form a straight line from shoulders to ankles, your stomach and glutes tight, and your chest open.

YOUR WEAKNESS: If you break form in any way, such as raising or dropping your hips, it means your entire core is weak, including your abs, glutes, and even your shoulders. To perfect your alignment, place a yardstick along your back so that during the plank it rests along your butt, upper back, and the back of your head. The best way to improve core strength? You guessed it. More planks. Start by holding for 20 to 30 seconds and build your endurance from there.

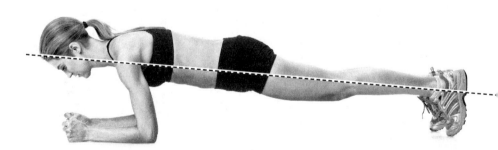

Side Plank Test

HOW TO DO IT: Lie on your left side with your knees straight. Prop your upper body up on your left elbow and forearm. Brace your core by contracting your abs forcefully. Raise your hips until your body forms a straight line from your ankles to your shoulders. Count for how many seconds you can hold this optimal alignment. Your eventual goal should be 30 seconds. Switch sides and repeat. Be sure to look for differences between your left and right sides.

SIDE VIEW

ASSESS YOUR FORM: How good is your alignment? Your body should be rigid, in a straight line. Your legs should be straight, your stomach and glutes tight, and your chest open.

YOUR WEAKNESS: If your hips sag or drift backward relative to your feet and torso, it means you may have a weakness in your obliques and trunk muscles. Strengthen these muscles with T-stabilizers (page 185).

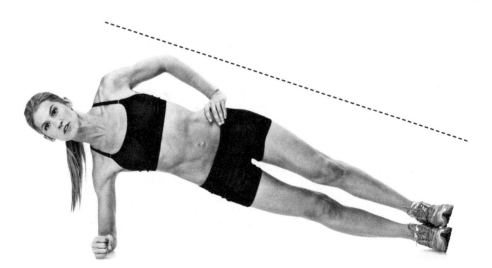

Perfect Your Posture

Even if you follow the *Women's Health* Fast-Track Tone-Up Plan to a T, you can't go back in time and eliminate years of hunching over a stair climber or all the time you spent slumped over your workstation, praying for the weekend to arrive. The day-to-day stresses literally change the shape of your alignment, which can leave you looking more hunchback than hottie. And over time, poor posture takes a tremendous toll on your spine, shoulders, hips, and knees. In fact, it can cause a cascade of structural flaws that result in acute problems, such as joint pain throughout your body, reduced flexibility, and compromised muscles, all of which can limit your ability to burn fat and build strength. Not good!

But don't worry—all these problems can be corrected. Are you ready to straighten yourself out? Use this head-to-toe guide to make sure your posture is picture-perfect.

Analyze Your Alignment

Wear something form-fitting and take two full-body photos, one from the front and one from the side. Relax your muscles but stand as tall as you can, with your feet hip-width apart. Now compare your photos to those at right to diagnose your posture problems. Notice the dotted line in the profile photo. Are your ear, hip, and ankle in alignment? If you spot one of the following problems, add our fixes to your regular workout plan.

DIAGNOSIS:

FORWARD HEAD

Your chin protrudes out from your chest and your legs are in front of your shoulders.

WHERE PAIN STRIKES: Neck

THE PROBLEM: Stiff muscles in the back of your neck

FIX IT: Stretch with head nods daily: Moving only your head, drop your chin down and in toward your neck while stretching the back of your neck. Hold for 5 seconds; do this 10 times.

THE PROBLEM: Weak muscles in front of your neck

FIX IT: Do this neck "crunch" every day: Lying faceup on the floor, lift your head so it just clears the floor. Raise your head and hold for 5 seconds; do 2 or 3 sets of 12 reps.

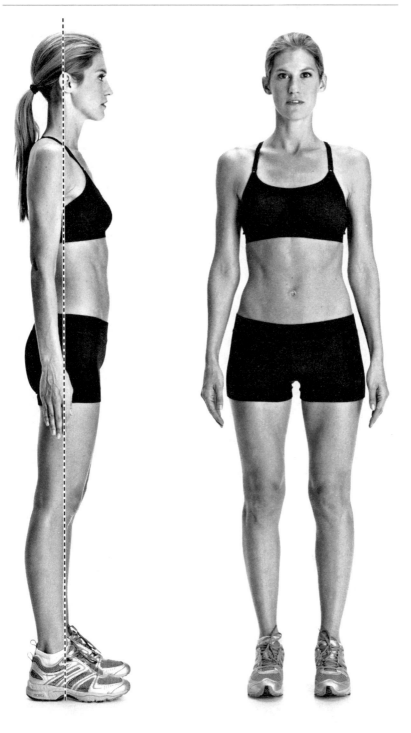

DIAGNOSIS:

ELEVATED SHOULDER

Your shoulders are not in line with your collar bone but encroach up toward your ears.

WHERE PAIN STRIKES: Neck and shoulders

THE PROBLEM: A shortened trapezius muscle (the muscle that starts at the back of your neck and runs across your upper back)

FIX IT: Perform an upper-trap stretch: With your higher-side arm behind your back, tilt your head away from your elevated side until you feel the stretch in your upper trapezius. Apply slight pressure with your free hand on your stretched muscle. Hold for 30 seconds; repeat 3 times.

THE PROBLEM: A weak serratus anterior, the muscle just under your pecs that runs from your upper ribs to your shoulder blades

FIX IT: Try chair shrugs. Sit upright in a chair with your hands next to your hips, palms down on the seat, and keep your arms straight. Without moving your arms, push down on the chair until your hips lift off the seat and your torso rises. Hold for 5 seconds. That's 1 rep; do 2 or 3 sets of 12 reps.

DIAGNOSIS:

ANTERIOR PELVIC TILT

Your lower abdomen protrudes forward and your lower back is arched.

WHERE PAIN STRIKES: Lower back (because of the more pronounced arch in your lumbar spine). The tilt also shifts your posture so that your stomach pushes outward, even if you don't have an ounce of belly fat.

THE PROBLEM: Tight hip flexors (muscles that allow you to move your thighs up to your abdomen)

FIX IT: Perform a front hip stretch: Kneel on one knee and tighten your gluteal (butt) muscles on your kneeling side until you feel the front of your hip stretching comfortably. Reach upward with the arm that's on your kneeling side and stretch in the opposite direction. Hold this position for a count of 30 seconds and repeat 3 times. Repeat the exercise on the other side.

THE PROBLEM: Weak glutes

FIX IT: The glute bridge is your solution: Lie on your back with your knees bent about 90 degrees. Squeeze your glutes together and push your hips upward until your body is straight from knees to shoulders. Hold for 5 seconds; complete 2 or 3 sets of 12 reps.

DIAGNOSIS:

ROUNDED SHOULDERS

Your shoulders are in front of your hips and ankles instead of in alignment with them.

WHERE PAIN STRIKES: Neck, shoulders, or back

THE PROBLEM: Tight pectoral (chest) muscles

FIX IT: Try a simple doorway stretch: Place your arms against a doorjamb in the high-five position (that is, forming an L), your elbow bent 90 degrees. Step through the doorway until you feel the stretch in your chest and the front of your shoulders. Hold for 30 seconds. That's 1 set; do a total of 4.

THE PROBLEM: Weakness in the middle and lower parts of your trapezius

FIX IT: Do the floor L-raise: Lying facedown on the floor, place each arm at a 90-degree angle in the high-five position. Without changing your elbow angle, raise both arms by pulling your shoulders back and squeezing your shoulder blades together. Hold for 5 seconds; do 2 or 3 sets of 12 reps.

DIAGNOSIS:

HUNCHED BACK

Your shoulders are rounded forward and your chest is concave.

WHERE PAIN STRIKES: Neck, shoulders, back

THE PROBLEM: Poor upper-back mobility

FIX IT: Lie faceup on a foam roller placed about midback, perpendicular to your spine. Place your hands behind your head and arch your upper back over the roller 5 times. Adjust the roller and repeat for each segment of your upper back.

THE PROBLEM: Weak muscles in your back

FIX IT: Perform the prone cobra: Lie facedown with your arms at your sides, palms down. Lift your chest and hands slightly off the floor, and squeeze your shoulder blades together while keeping your chin down. Hold for 5 seconds; do 2 or 3 sets of 12 reps.

DIAGNOSIS:

PIGEON TOES

One or both feet point slightly inward instead of straight ahead.

WHERE PAIN STRIKES: Knee, hip, or lower back

THE PROBLEM: Tightness in the outer portion of your thigh (your tensor fasciae latae)

FIX IT: Stand up, cross your affected leg behind the other, and lean away from the affected side until you feel your hip stretching comfortably. Hold for 30 seconds. Repeat 3 times.

THE PROBLEM: Weak gluteus maximus and medius muscles

FIX IT: Use an exercise called the side-lying clamshell: Lie on one side with your knees bent 90 degrees and your heels together. Keeping your hips still, raise your top knee upward, separating your knees like a clamshell. Pause for 5 seconds; lower your knee to the starting position. Perform 2 or 3 sets of 12 reps. Repeat on the other side.

DIAGNOSIS:

DUCK FEET

One or both feet point slightly outward instead of straight ahead.

WHERE PAIN STRIKES: Hip or lower back

THE PROBLEM: A lack of flexibility in your hip muscles.

FIX IT: Drop to your hands | and knees and place one foot behind the opposite knee. Making sure you keep your spine naturally arched, shift your weight backward and allow your hips to bend until you feel the stretch. Hold the stretch for 30 seconds, repeat 3 times, and then switch sides.

THE PROBLEM: Weakness in your oblique muscles and hip flexors

FIX IT: Try the Swiss-ball jackknife: Assume the top of a pushup position but rest your feet on a Swiss ball. Without rounding your lower back, tuck your knees under your torso by rolling the ball with your feet toward your body. Roll the ball back to the starting position. Do 2 or 3 sets of 12 reps daily.

You can't go from
flab to fab unless
you choose the right
exercises that burn
the most fat.

3

THE FEMALE BODY AT 20, 30, 40, AND BEYOND!

Everything you need to know about your body—right now and for the future.

Each and every day of her life, a woman makes thousands of decisions. What will I eat for breakfast? What errands should I run on my lunch break? The gym after work or happy hour at 6? *Grey's* on the DVR or a good night's sleep?

Few of these decisions will change the course of your life. But day by day, those choices add up to a pattern, a pattern that will reveal itself as the years pass, the way crop circles become apparent when you get up in altitude. By the time a woman is in her mid-thirties, those decisions may have shaped her into a classic combo of youth, grace, and style like Eva Longoria or an off-the-rails hot mess like Tara Reid (both born in 1975). By the time she's in her late forties, day-to-day choices will determine whether she looks more like the always-elegant Sandra Bullock or the Botoxed and bloated Courtney Love (both born circa 1964). When that same woman is closing in on 60, she may resemble perennial pinup Christie Brinkley or be dowdy and doughy like Kathleen Turner (both born in 1954).

You know which of those women you'd want to look like. You don't want to resemble the one who used to have her act together, who used to be a star, who used to be sexy. You want to be a woman who still is those things—at any age.

Well, you can be.

It starts with giving well-deserved attention to your health, nutrition, and fitness. It's hard to maintain your edge when all your edges have gone soft, after all. The *Women's Health* Nutrition System and the *Women's Health* Fast-Track Tone-Up Plan are calibrated to strip away fat—starting with your belly first—no matter your age, or how long that extra weight has been hanging around causing trouble.

But a lot of the battle is also about understanding how your body changes over the first few decades of adulthood and making adjustments in your health and fitness routines so you have the tools you

> **HOT TIP #30**
>
> **See your way to the gym.** You'll cut your risk of age-related macular degeneration—the leading cause of adult blindness—by 70 percent simply by exercising three times a week, according to a University of Wisconsin study.

need to carry you into your later years. No matter how fit you are, a health crisis at any point can undermine your best-laid plans. *Women's Health* talked to the world's leading cardiologists, neuroscientists, nutritionists, and trainers to create this guide to your twenties, thirties, forties, and beyond. It will help you anticipate your body's physiological shifts and then guide you through critical adjustments to your lifestyle to match them.

HOT TIP #31

Order off the menu. Most restaurants have healthier choices—brown rice instead of white—that aren't listed on the daily menu. Don't be afraid to ask if there's something better hiding in the kitchen.

Yes, you will grow older, but you will also grow sexier, stronger, and even smarter. Here's what you need to know in order to work these changes to your advantage and build the best body you can, no matter what your age.

Your Twenties

Your Muscles

In your twenties, your body has the ability to handle intense frequent exercise, says Alexander Koch, PhD, an associate professor of exercise sciences at Truman State University, in Missouri. The reason: Levels of testosterone (yes, you have this hormone) and human growth hormone—both of which spur growth of the muscle fibers that power intense activities—are at their highest. No matter what your age or gender, developing lean muscle is like putting money in the bank: It will help keep your metabolism high in the coming years, fending off weight gain and lowering your diabetes risk. (And, no, it won't bulk you up into the Incredible Hulk.) Plus, it will protect you against injury. But as with money, the earlier you can bank it, the greater the long-term payoff.

YOUR PLAN: To make the most muscle gains while strength training, switch up your reps every 2 to 4 weeks, or even every workout. Arizona State University researchers discovered that people who alternated their rep ranges—a technique called undulating periodization—in each of three weekly training sessions gained twice as much strength as those who did the same number of reps every workout.

HOT TIP #32

Write it down.
In a 13-week study, dieters who kept a food record for 3 weeks or longer lost 3.5 pounds more than those who didn't, say researchers at the University of Arkansas. To eyeball calories like an expert, log your daily meals for at least 2 weeks on a free Web site like sparkpeople.com.

Your Skin

This is a fairly maintenance-free decade, says David Bank, MD, a dermatologist in Mount Kisco, New York. Your skin still has plenty of elastin (the protein that helps skin spring back after stretching) and collagen (the fibrous structural protein that keeps tissue plump).

YOUR PLAN: The bulk of future wrinkles and sun discolorations are earned before and during this decade, so protect yourself with sunscreen of at least SPF 30, says Rebecca Giles, MD, the owner of FIX skin clinic in Malibu, California. Look for broad-spectrum protection against UVA and UVB rays; products with titanium and zinc oxide block both. A great way to remember to use it: Put it on every day along with moisturizer.

Your Stress Level

Thanks to a smorgasbord of twentysomething stressors—the kind that come with 70-hour workweeks and late nights on the cocktail circuit—the first episodes of depression often hit women in their twenties. But it's not just your mind that pays the price. A busy, high-stress lifestyle often leads to a diet of convenience—one that's lacking in vitamins and minerals and is overloaded with sugar, fat, and calories. The result: a body that never realizes its full potential.

YOUR PLAN: Eat 1 tablespoon of ground flaxseed daily. It's the best source of alpha-linolenic acid, or ALA—a healthy fat that improves the workings of the cerebral cortex, the area of the brain that processes sensory information, including that of pleasure, says Jean Marie Bourre, PhD, a nutrition researcher at Hôpital Fernand Widal, in Paris. Find ground flaxseed in the health food section of your grocery store. To meet your quota, sprinkle it on salads, vegetables, and cereal or mix it in a yogurt, smoothie or shake.

Your Cancer Risk

Every hour, your body replicates 6 billion cells, creating copies of your DNA. But if you don't consume enough folate—a B vitamin that helps construct those cells—your body could produce irregular DNA, which can eventually cause cancer, says Ann Yelmokas McDermott, PhD, MS, a nutrition scientist at Tufts University. Trouble is, folate is hard to come by. The best natural food source is chicken liver (yuck), and few women get the folate their bodies require from fruits and vegetables.

YOUR PLAN: The *Women's Health* Nutrition System is designed to boost your intake of vegetables and beans, and hence folate. But as a backup plan, have a cup of folate-fortified cereal 4 days a week. Choose a brand that provides at least 400 micrograms of folate per serving—such as Total Raisin Bran or Multi-Grain Cheerios. Then top it with cup of blackberries, raspberries, or strawber-

> **HOT TIP #33**
>
> **Build it with badminton.**
> Swedish scientists discovered that badminton players saw greater increases in bone density than ice hockey players. Why? In badminton, about 15 percent of your moves are lunges, meaning you're working the large muscles in the legs, crucial for bone-building.

ries. Berries aren't just a good nonliver source of folate; they're also packed with antioxidants, which help thwart cancer by neu-tralizing DNA-damaging free radicals.

Your Bones

Bones are a lot like reclusive coworkers; until one snaps, you aren't likely to give it much thought. But this is your last chance to lay down new bone; by the time you're 30, your skeletal system is set.

Super-Quick Health Fixes

These simple changes will improve, prolong, and even save your life

WHEN: Before dinner
THE CHANGE: Have a snack.
THE BENEFIT: A 4-pound weight loss in a year. Eating ½ ounce of a healthy fat, like nuts or avocado, 8 minutes before a meal keeps you satis-fied for 3 hours, com-pared with 20 minutes without. As a result, you eat less, says Michael Roizen, MD, a professor at Upstate Medical University, in New York.

WHEN: At happy hour
THE CHANGE: Drink red wine from Chile instead of France.
THE BENEFIT: Reduced risk of cancer. Chilean cabernet sauvignon is 38 percent higher in flavonol (an antiox-idant that fights can-cer-causing cells) than French wine.

WHEN: At dessert
THE CHANGE: Substitute a Fudgsi-cle for your daily Hershey bar.
THE BENEFIT: A 10-pound weight loss over a year. You'll save 100 calories every night

WHEN: At work
THE CHANGE: Walk to your coworker's desk instead of sending an e-mail.
THE BENEFIT: More than 1 pound of weight loss a year through the added calorie burn. Plus, one study showed that walking an extra 4,000 to 5,000 steps a day could reduce your blood pressure by 11 points.

WHEN: With every meal
THE CHANGE: Drink ice water.

Poor nutrition not only inhibits your ability to grow bone; it also increases your both—risk of gaining weight and a whole host of other medical problems now and for decades down the road.

YOUR PLAN: Drink two 8-ounce glasses of vitamin D–fortified milk every day. This provides your body with 600 milligrams of calcium and 5 micrograms of vitamin D, the perfect combination of nutrients to build break-resistant bones. Broccoli also deserves a place on your menu. It contains a respectable 45 milligrams of calcium

THE BENEFIT: A pound lost every 8 weeks, if you make it eight 8-ounce glasses a day. You'll expend 123 calories of heat daily to warm the water to 98.6 degrees Fahrenheit.

WHEN: When you get out of bed
THE CHANGE: Stand up and stretch your hamstrings for 30 seconds.
THE BENEFIT: A 27 percent increase in flexibility in 6 weeks.

WHEN: At lunch
THE CHANGE: Swap your ham sandwich for tuna.
THE BENEFIT: An 8 percent reduced risk of heart disease. The

omega-3 fatty acids in fish have been found to help raise your good cholesterol and keep your arteries clean.

WHEN: After your workout
THE CHANGE: Drink a postworkout chocolate milk.
THE BENEFIT: Muscle recovery and growth. A University of Washington study found that drinks that blend carbohydrates and protein, such as chocolate milk, are nearly 40 percent more effective than protein alone at helping your muscles recover and grow after a workout.

WHEN: Before you brush your teeth
THE CHANGE: Take one regular aspirin.
THE BENEFIT: 20 percent reduced risk of breast cancer. Studies show that women who take one aspirin a day have a 20 percent lower incidence of breast cancer.

WHEN: Before bed
THE CHANGE: Have a piece of chocolate.
THE BENEFIT: Better sex. One study showed that women who ate chocolate reported more satisfying sex lives than those who didn't.

per cup, along with magnesium, vitamin K, and phosphorus, all of which, research shows, play a major role in keeping you upright from here to Social Security.

Your Cervix

Cervical cancer is the fourth-most-common form of the disease in women ages 20 to 39. It also has one of the highest survival rates: more than 90 percent, according to the American Cancer Society. Of course, you have to catch it first, and because the early signs are not visible to the naked eye, it's critical that you get tested regularly.

YOUR PLAN: The American College of Obstetrics and Gynecology now says that women should get their first Pap smear, which tests for precancerous changes that are usually caused by human papilloma viruses (HPV), at age 21, with follow-up tests every other year until they turn 30. Women over 30 who have had three consecutive "normal" results can then wait 3 years between tests. The group points to studies showing that only 0.1 percent of cervical cancer cases occur in women under 21, but that does little to ease worries that the disease could grow undetected between spaced out exams. The bottom line: "It's all about risk," says Celeste Robb Nicholson, MD, associate chief of general medicine at Massachusetts General Hospital. "A healthy woman who is HPV-negative and either is not sexually active or has just one partner can be screened every 3 years. Women who have risk factors—such as smoking and having multiple partners—should be screened annually."

Also talk to your ob-gyn about the cervical cancer vaccine, which is effective against four virus strains, including two that cause about 70 percent of cervical cancers.

> **HOT TIP #34**
>
> **Mate (again and again) for life.**
> A study of 1,000 middle-age subjects found that those who had frequent orgasms had a 50 percent lower death rate. Can we get a prescription for that?

Your HIV Status

Of the estimated 1 million Americans infected with HIV, 25 percent don't know they're infected, so they aren't taking medicines to suppress it, according to the Centers for Disease Control and Prevention. That's why the CDC recommends that everyone—even those in low-risk groups—be screened routinely for the disease.

YOUR PLAN: The best screening is the two-part HIV ELISA/Western blot test. The HIV ELISA (enzyme-linked immunosorbent assay) requires a blood sample, but oral swabs are an option for the needlephobic. The second test, the Western blot, is needed to confirm the ELISA results, because other conditions, such as lupus, Lyme disease, and syphilis, can produce a false-positive ELISA result. The FDA has also approved a do-it-yourself kit called Home Access HIV-1, which allows you to send a prick of blood to a private lab for confidential testing.

HOT TIP #35

Listen to smoothie jazz. Whey protein not only helps you build muscle, but it boosts your body's production of glutathione, an antioxidant that University of Buffalo researchers found could limit noise-induced hearing loss in mice.

Your Blood Sugar

The American Diabetes Association estimates that one-third of US adults with type 2 diabetes don't know they have it. What's more, most of them could have avoided the condition altogether through preventive screening. "If your fasting blood glucose is in a prediabetic range [between 100 and 125 milligrams per deciliter], you can prevent the disease with lifestyle changes," says David Johnson, PhD, coauthor of *Medical Tests That Can Save Your Life*.

YOUR PLAN: A study in the *New England Journal of Medicine* found that if you have prediabetes, exercising for 30 minutes a day and losing 5 percent of your body weight through a diet rich in fruits, vegetables, and fiber could reduce your risk of developing diabetes by 58 percent. You should get a fasting blood glucose test once a year, starting in your twenties.

Your Teeth

There's a strong link between periodontal disease and blood markers for heart disease. When oral bacteria travel through the bloodstream, they can cause the liver to pump out C-reactive protein (CRP), high levels of which indicate inflammation, says Brent Bauer, MD, associate professor of medicine at the Mayo Clinic. "That inflammation may be a factor in causing atherosclerosis," or the buildup of cholesterol and other fatty materials on your artery all. Fortunately, gum disease is usually reversible if caught early.

YOUR PLAN: Get a dental exam and cleaning twice a year.

HOT TIP #36

Prolong your workout. When you're in the middle of a run or bike ride, and you feel like hanging it up, take a deep breath and blow out hard. This mind-clearing technique is known as the "explosive exhale." It allows you to "blow out all your demons," says Amby Burfoot, former Boston Marathon champion and contributing editor of *Runner's World*.

Your Belly

Sixty-four percent of American women are overweight or obese, but only 5 percent recognize that they have a problem, according to a recent Pew Research Survey. Ignorance can be deadly. Obesity is linked to a number of diseases, including high blood pressure, diabetes, heart disease, and even cancer.

YOUR PLAN: Use the body mass index, which estimates body fat based on your height and weight, to determine if you're in the danger zone (visit womenshealthmag.com/files/bmi-calculator/index.html for a calculator). Measure yourself every 3 years or whenever you gain weight, starting in your twenties. A score between 18.5 and 24.9 is normal. BMI doesn't take into account muscle mass, though, so if you work out with weights often (as you should), use the US Navy circumference method (go to dietandfitnesstoday.com/bodyfat.php). You'll need to take a few measurements, but you'll get a more accurate reading.

HOT TIP #37

Pop one for productivity. Taking a multivitamin could make you a better multitasker, say UK researchers. Try a multi with a 300 percent daily value (DV) of vitamin B6, 150 percent DV of folic acid, and 50 percent DV of vitamin B12.

Your Life

According to the CDC, "unintentional injuries" are the number-one cause of death for women in their twenties. Car crashes are the leading cause of accidental death among otherwise healthy young women and, of those, the number caused by driver inattention has risen 21 percent in the past 5 years.

YOUR PLAN: Stop multitasking while driving: Turn off your cell phone, save your snacks for later, and never, ever apply makeup behind the wheel (20 percent of women admit doing it!).

Your Thirties

Your Muscles

You may find that you don't recover as quickly from a workout as you did in your twenties. Testosterone and growth hormones that assist recovery start to decline once you hit the big 3-0. In fact, researchers have found that these hormones decline more dramatically in your reproductive years than they do after menopause, according to a study in the *Journal of Clinical Endocrinology and Metabolism*. Bottom line: It will take longer for your muscles to return to full strength after each sweat session.

YOUR PLAN: Eat broccoli and bell peppers. Together, they're packed with vitamins C and E, two nutrients that fight free radicals—rogue molecules that slow the repair of exercise-induced muscle damage, impeding recovery.

> **HOT TIP #38**
>
> **Mix and max.**
> To maximize gains, vary reps and the amount of weight you lift. Muscles grow when they are forced to adapt. A recent study in the *Journal of Strength and Conditioning Research* found that people who regularly varied their reps increased their bench strength by 28 percent and their leg-press strength by 43 percent.

Your Skin

This is a transitional decade for your skin. You've kind of passed your peak oil moment, face-wise: Oil production drops about 10 percent in this decade, and the skin thins about the same amount. Prior sun damage begins to crop up in the form of crow's-feet and furrows in your forehead, and skin starts to sag, thanks to collagen loss. A late night is far more likely to bring out dark circles, bags, and puffiness.

YOUR PLAN: If you like to work out al fresco, try to schedule exercise before 10 a.m. or after 4 p.m. Sweat breaks down the skin's defenses and allow more ultraviolet light and pollutants to reach skin cells. If you can stay out of the sunlight in the late morning and early afternoon, you can avoid the most damaging UVB rays. And remember, you don't have to be Lady Gaga to wear a splashy hat with a brim, especially on clear summer days.

Your Metabolism

The metabolic rate that allowed you to burn through late-night postdrinking diner trips in your twenties is now dropping slowly but surely. Research shows that starting at age 30, you will lose 10 percent of the total muscle on your body over the next 20 years.

And even if the number on your scale isn't rising, the size of your little black dress probably is.

YOUR PLAN: Hit the weights. A study in the *American Journal of Clinical Nutrition* found that even people who did not gain weight for 38 years lost 3 pounds of muscle and added 3 pounds of fat each decade. Regular resistance training can help you avoid this fate.

Your Joints

Even though arthritis doesn't usually set in until later in life, the damage that causes it, cartilage degeneration, is happening now.

YOUR PLAN: Eat three 6-ounce servings of cold-water fish weekly. Specifically, have salmon, mackerel, trout, or white tuna; each packs more than 1,000 milligrams of fish oil. A UK study found that regularly consuming this amount of fish oil appeared to halt cartilage-eating enzymes in 86 percent of people who are facing joint-replacement surgery. Fish oil slows down cartilage degeneration and reduces factors that cause inflammation, says lead researcher Bruce Caterson, PhD.

Your Blood Pressure

Starting at age 30, your systolic blood pressure rises 4 points per decade. Researchers from the Netherlands recently discovered that besides the obvious factors—obesity, lack of physical activity, and high salt consumption—diets containing too little potassium were the primary cause of hypertension. In their analysis, the scientists used 3,500 milligrams daily as the cutoff for defining a "low" potassium intake. That's bad news, because the average American woman in her thirties gets only about 2,500 milligrams a day.

> **HOT TIP #39**
>
> **Pencil it in.**
> Schedule your workout like you schedule any other meetings. If you make appointments for meetings and business lunches, schedule your gym time as well.

YOUR PLAN: Include ½ cup of beans, a banana, and a handful of raisins in your daily diet. Each will increase your potassium intake by about 400 milligrams a day. And don't forget to test your blood pressure once a year. A reading below 120/80 millimeters of mercury is desirable, and anything over 140/90 mmHg is cause for concern. If you fall in that middle zone (between 120/80 and 139/89 mmHg), take note: You have prehypertension, which means you're likely to develop high blood pressure if you don't start taking preventive action now.

> **HOT TIP #40**
>
> **Tag-team your weight loss.**
> Work out with a friend and you'll exercise for an additional 34 minutes, according to the American College of Sports Medicine. And researchers at the University of Oxford found that exercisers who trained in a group tolerated pain better than those who exercised alone.

Your Heart

Fifty percent of heart attacks occur in people with normal levels of LDL cholesterol (the bad kind), so if you're in a high-risk group because of race, blood pressure, or family history, you might benefit from asking your doctor for some additional blood tests.

YOUR PLAN: The high-sensitivity CRP test looks for elevated levels of C-reactive protein, which is produced by your liver in response to inflammation and is as predictive of heart disease as high cholesterol. Elevated levels of the amino acid homocysteine often signal the buildup of plaque, cholesterol, and calcium in your arteries, says Stanley Hazen, MD, PhD, director of the Cleveland Clinic's Center for Cardiovascular Diagnostics and Prevention. At least once every 5 years, starting in your twenties, you should have a full lipid profile test. Unlike common cholesterol screens, this blood test measures the levels of four different kinds of blood fats: LDL cholesterol, HDL cholesterol, very low-density lipoprotein (VLDL), and triglycerides. It provides a clearer picture of circulatory health and helps your physician pinpoint any problems, says Thomas Owens, MD, of Duke University Medical Center.

Your Sex Drive

You're climbing the company ladder, maybe getting married and having kids, dealing with a mother-in-law, a 401(k), a mortgage . . . you're stretched and stressed to your limits. Oh yeah, and your sex life is about as revved up as a rusty tractor.

YOUR PLAN: Go nuts. Peanuts, hazelnuts, and walnuts are loaded with vitamin E, an antioxidant that bolsters the immune system, which gets down when you're running around. Bonus: Nuts are also a great food source of arginine, an amino acid that improves blood flow—to help you get from dead tired to orgasmic. You need only a handful per day, so sprinkle them on yogurt, salads, or oatmeal—or just snack on them plain.

Your Belly

From your thirties on, you start to add on the adipose (a.k.a. flab). Your metabolism slows and your body-fat percentage creeps up. But more than any other measure, your body-fat percentage indicates your overall health.

YOUR PLAN: Work to keep your BMI, your body mass index, between 18.5 and 24.9; research shows that doing this reduces your risk of high blood pressure, diabetes, and heart disease. Eating the right breakfast will keep your belly at bay, according to multiple studies of the sub-

HOT TIP #41

Sleep or work out?
Sleep! "If you're sleep deprived and not just groggy, stay in bed," says Alan Aragon, MS, a nutritionist in Thousand Oaks, California. University of Chicago researchers found that lack of sleep packs on pounds by slowing metabolism and increasing your appetite.

ject. Filling it with protein is key: People on weight-loss diets who break eggs for breakfast, for instance, lose 65 percent more weight than those who down a bagel with the same number of calories, according to a study in the *International Journal of Obesity*.

Your Back

HOT TIP #42

Get sex on the brain. Regular romps in the sack might make your brain grow. Sexually active lab rats showed spikes in brain cells and neurons in the hippocampus, the area responsible for memory and learning, according to a study published in PLoS ONE. (Too bad they didn't use human volunteers.)

More than 50 percent of women in their thirties suffer from lower-back pain, and that number rises to nearly 70 percent during pregnancy.

YOUR PLAN: Shore up your core. Do the side bridge three times a week. Lie on your left side with knees straight and upper body propped on your left elbow and forearm. Place your right hand on your right hip and slowly raise your hips until your body forms a straight line from your shoulders to your knees. Hold for 5 to 10 seconds, breathing deeply. That's one rep. Repeat four times, then switch to your right side. Do one to two sets on each side. Too hard? Bend your knees 90 degrees so that they rest on the floor. If you're pregnant, do the exercise with your back against a wall for support.

Your Stress Level

All those stressors we mentioned earlier? They affect more than your sex drive. They cause levels of the stress hormone cortisol go up. Cortisol is also the belly-fat hormone: It can actually blunt the body's production of testosterone (yes, even in women) and cause your belly to bulge.

YOUR PLAN: Find something to laugh at. Even the anticipation of a good laugh decreases the stress chemicals cortisol and epinephrine by 39 and 70 percent, respectively, say researchers at Loma Linda University. Laughter is also great for the heart. When participants in a University of Maryland study watched stressful film clips, they experienced vasoconstriction, a narrowing of the blood vessels. But the blood vessels of those watching funny films expanded by 22 percent.

HOT TIP #43

Don't drain in vain. The clear liquid on the top of yogurt is pure whey protein—the stuff they charge you $5 a pop for at the gym. Don't drain it off, just stir it back in and enjoy.

Your Forties & Beyond

Your Libido

It's more lifeless than a dorm-room houseplant. In your forties, hormonal changes and stress (still, ugh!) can cause your desire to lag. In particular, the hormone testosterone—which, combined

How Fast Are You Aging?

Use these five simple tests to find out if time is taking its toll… and what you can do to set back the clock.

MUSCLE MASS

THE TEST: Stand with your feet shoulder-width apart. Keeping your back straight and shoulders square, drop into a sitting position and rise back up in one fluid motion. You should be able to do eight of these unweighted squat exercises and also one pushup with good form (meaning your body stays in a straight line from head to toe as you lower it to the floor and raise it back up). For more fitness tests (and solutions), see Chapters 2 and 8.

SIGNS OF A PROBLEM: Sarcopenia, the age-related loss of muscle mass, progresses slowly and almost imperceptibly. If you can't do eight squats or one good pushup, you need to rebuild your strength.

WHAT TO DO: Incorporate 30 minutes of resistance training into your routine at least 2 days a week. Try lunges, bicep curls, and tricep pushdowns. The *Women's Health* Fast-Track Tone-Up Plan is designed to help you build new muscle while burning off excess flab.

HEARING

THE TEST: Go to freemosquitoringtones.org and give yourself the age-appropriate test.

SIGNS OF A PROBLEM: If certain consonants, such as C, D, K, P, S, and T, become hard to distinguish, see a hearing specialist.

WHAT TO DO: Eat lean meat, fish, poultry, eggs, and dairy—all high in vitamin B_{12}—and folate-rich leafy green vegetables, citrus fruits, and beans. Lack of these vitamins has been linked to age-related hearing loss.

with estrogen, fuels your sex drive—starts to decline right about now. Testosterone levels are also affected by oral contraceptives. **YOUR PLAN:** If your lust levels plummet after going on the Pill, switch to condoms or try an IUD. Otherwise, if your sex drive is sluggish, have your hormone levels checked and work with an endocrinologist to make sure you're getting enough testosterone.

EYESIGHT

THE TEST: How far away do you hold a book when reading? It should be less than an arm's length away. **SIGNS OF A PROBLEM:** If you're holding your reading material farther away than usual, it is a sign of age-related vision loss. **WHAT TO DO:** When reading, make sure that you have sufficient light so you aren't straining to see. Eat carrots, spinach, and kale, all of which are high in vitamin A and lutein, two essential vitamins for maintaining healthy vision. And go to an optometrist for further testing if your eyes tire easily.

MEMORY

THE TEST: You should be able to remember up to seven random numbers after seeing them for only 3 seconds. **SIGNS OF A PROBLEM:** Forgetting the name of someone you just met or where you put your keys is normal. Not recognizing a family member or knowing what your keys are used for are signs of a more serious problem. **WHAT TO DO:** Challenge your brain with puzzles, stay physically active, and go out often with your friends. All of these activities have been shown to keep people mentally sharp.

BALANCE

THE TEST: Close your eyes, stand on one leg, and hold the knee of your raised leg close to your chest for 30 seconds. You should be able to do this without dropping the raised leg or hopping around. **SIGNS OF A PROBLEM:** If you trip, slip, and bump into things on a daily basis, or notice that you often feel dizzy or lightheaded, you should see a doctor. **WHAT TO DO:** Tai chi or yoga will improve muscle coordination and blood circulation while increasing muscle strength and tone.

Your Muscles

Your body is still shedding muscle—in fact, by the time you reach 40, you're losing about 0.5 percent of your muscle mass every year. And a lot of that comes simply from neglect—skipping the gym literally causes you to replace muscle with fat, according to a *Journal of the American College of Nutrition* study. That's particularly problematic, because a pound of fat takes up more space on your body than a pound of muscle. So even if you weigh the same as you did on your wedding day, you may not be as shapely as you once were.

YOUR PLAN: In addition to lifting weights, you can protect your hard-earned muscles by feeding them the right foods. Ounce for ounce, tuna is one of the best sources of muscle-boosting protein—and contains zero saturated fat. Spinach can help with muscle maintenance; recent test-tube research from Rutgers University found that a hormone in spinach increases protein synthesis. Spinach is also rich in vitamin K, potassium, and calcium, which can help you ward off osteoporosis.

> **HOT TIP #44**
>
> **Drop weight by raisin it.** The raisins in commercial raisin brans are typically coated with sugar. Buy wheat flakes and add your own dried fruits. You'll save 7 grams of sugar— enough to lose 5 pounds in a year if you do it every day.

Your Joints

Your nerve fibers are losing their effectiveness, which diminishes coordination. Your heart beats more slowly, cutting down the blood flow that delivers nutrients to and removes waste from joints and muscles. As a result, those key body parts that are so essential to smooth motion—wrists, elbows, knees, ankles—are becoming more vulnerable to injury and to the onset of arthritis.

YOUR PLAN: Your workouts should emphasize flexibility. New science shows that doing yoga can improve flexibility, relieve back pain, and reduce stress. Boston University researchers report that people who did yoga weekly boosted levels of the antianxiety brain chemical GABA by 27 percent. Practicing yoga can also help your body maintain its antioxidant levels, which deplete when you're run down, report Indian researchers.

Your Wrinkles

In your forties, crow's-feet become permanent creases, and expression lines on your forehead are more difficult to ignore. The loss of tissue under the eyes may produce a hollow look. Moisture production drops another 10 percent, and collagen continues to plummet, causing additional wrinkles to form.

YOUR PLAN: Soothe parched skin with extra emollients overnight. Look for a night cream that lists one of these active ingredients: retinol (vitamin A), antioxidants, vitamin C, or peptides.

Your Skin

After all those years you spent soaking up the rays covered by nothing but a string bikini and a thin coating of SPF 2, it's payback time. Now is the time when previous sun damage can get dangerous. The most important thing is to catch anything potentially cancerous early so it can be removed.

YOUR PLAN: Examine your freckles and sunspots, birthmarks and moles, making sure to look for the ABCDs: Asymmetrical; Borders with ragged edges; Color changes; or Diameters bigger than 6 millimeters. If you've spent a lot of time in the sun or gone 5 years without a professional exam, ask your doctor, preferably a dermatologist, to look you over. Mutating moles are

HOT TIP #45

Gobble more. Substituting turkey for beef or pork slashes an average of 108 calories per meal.

scary, but certain foods can help: National Cancer Institute researchers determined that people with a high intake of carotenoids—pigments that occur naturally in plants—were as much as six times less likely to develop skin cancer than those with a low intake. Eat two servings of sweet potatoes, carrots, or cantaloupe every week.

Your Vision

Even if your peepers are still twenty-twenty, two eye conditions that can lead to vision loss—cataracts and macular degeneration—can start to develop during this time. (And women are at higher risk for macular degeneration than men.)

YOUR PLAN: The National Institutes of Health found that people who consume the most lutein—a carotenoid found in plant foods—are 43 percent less likely to develop macular degeneration. Lutein helps filter blue light, preventing it from damaging retinal tissues. Eat two servings of greens each day. Consider one serving to be ½ cup of cooked spinach, broccoli, or brussels sprouts. And, once every 2 years get a glaucoma test (also known as a tonometry), because more than 1 million women over 40 develop the most common form of glaucoma, according to the National Eye Institute. A simple eye exam—which looks for symptoms such as increased eye pressure and general vision deterioration—is all it takes to catch the disease early.

> **HOT TIP #46**
>
> **Go into the light.** Exercising in direct sunlight helps you lose up to 20 percent more body fat by boosting the appetite-killing hormone leptin.

Your Breasts

Your chances of getting breast cancer increase drastically as you get older—in fact, according to the American Cancer Society, between 2002 and 2006, 95 percent of new cases and 97 percent of breast cancer deaths occurred in women 40 and older.

YOUR PLAN: A low-fat diet can reduce your risk, but for even more protection, add cruciferous vegetables, such as broccoli and kale, to your plate. They contain sulforaphane, which is believed to help prevent cancer cells from multiplying. Johns Hopkins University researchers discovered that broccoli sprouts (baby broccoli) have up to 20 times as much of this compound as fully grown plants.

It's also a good idea to become familiar with the normal changes of your breasts by examining them monthly, in the days just after your period. For instructions, visit mayoclinic.com. As for screening, the American Cancer Society has long held that women should have their first annual mammogram at age 40, but recommendations released by the US Preventive Services Task Force in 2009 say most don't need them until they turn 50. The reason? Younger, denser breasts are more likely to produce benign cysts, and aggressive testing on innocent lumps is expensive and emotionally unsettling. Some doctors are sticking with earlier screenings until studies prove that fewer exams won't equal higher fatalities. The bottom line: Get tested annually starting at age 40, or earlier if you have a family history of breast cancer. Start screenings 10 years earlier than the age of your relative at the time of her diagnosis (so if your mom was diagnosed at age 42, for example, you should have your first mammogram at 32).

> **HOT TIP #47**
>
> **Be wind blown.** When you're cycling or running, start out with the wind behind you and return facing the wind. This way you get a boost when you're cold. Wind in your face is more tolerable once you've warmed up.

Your Heart

Until age 44, accidents are the most likely cause of death in women. But once you reach 45, heart disease becomes second only to cancer as your number-one threat. At age 40 and older, 23 percent of women will die within one year after a heart attack, compared with 18 percent of men.

YOUR PLAN: With proper conditioning (high-intensity activities such as circuit training work best), you can increase your heart's stroke volume and your body's oxygen uptake. This allows your heart to pump blood more slowly and efficiently, and that increases your longevity. It all comes down to how many times your heart beats before it conks out. "The average human life span is about 3 billion heartbeats," says Michael Lauer, MD, of the National Heart, Blood, and Lung Institute. "If you can lower your heart rate, you can increase your life expectancy." It's that simple. (The *Women's Health* Fast-Track Tone-Up Plan will raise your heart rate into the aerobic zone, helping you to strengthen your ticker right along with the rest of your body.) If you have a family history of heart disease, consider getting a 64-slice CT scan once at the age of 40, then every 5 years or as necessary, depending on the results. The scan is able to record images so fast that it captures your heart between beats and renders it in 3-D, providing a clearer picture of your coronary arteries than any other type of scan. It detects hard and soft plaques on arterial walls and gauges your risk of having a heart attack in the future.

> **HOT TIP #48**
>
> **Count backward.**
> When you're counting repetitions, start with your target number and count backward—you'll be thinking how few you have left instead of how many you've done.

Your Stroke Risk

Strokes are the third-leading cause of death in the United States. Eighty percent of all strokes are due to blood clots caused by plaque, and half the time, your first symptom is your last.

YOUR PLAN: Consider getting a carotid duplex ultrasound once at age 40, then as necessary, depending on the results. This noninvasive 10-minute test could show if you're at risk. It provides two views of the arteries in your neck, which reveal damage from plaque buildup and how that damage is affecting blood flow to your brain. This test isn't normally covered by insurance, but you can get it for less than $100 from a handful of private companies.

Your Colon

Colon cancer is the third-most-common type of cancer among women and the third-leading cause of cancer-related death, but many women have never been screened for it. There's good reason to catch it early: The survival rate is 93 percent if the cancer is treated before it spreads beyond the colon's walls.

YOUR PLAN: Of all the tests used to screen for colon cancer, the colonoscopy is the gold standard. The problem with most other tests is that either they don't examine the colon directly (the fecal occult blood test, for example, analyzes your stool for blood) or they don't reach far enough inside your colon (in the case of a slightly less invasive procedure known as a sigmoidscopy). It's a big organ, and 50 percent of all colon cancers occur in the half that's not examined by a sigmoidoscope. A colonoscopy, however, examines every inch, right up to the small intestine. If there's a history of colorectal cancer in your family, schedule this test about 10 years earlier than the age of your relative when he or she was first diagnosed, or in your early forties.

HOT TIP #49

Take tea for teeth. Researchers in Japan assessed the drinking habits of some 25,000 adults and found that those who drank at least a cup of green tea a day had a lower risk of tooth loss than those who drank none.

A MATTER OF FAT
Five reasons that
belly won't budge

Where does fat come from? And why do we have it? We'll reveal the nutritional and kinesiological science behind your gut and explain why it can be so damaging to your health. And we'll examine the surprising role that modern science plays in making us fat.

Saddlebags, spare tires, muffin tops—we've dreamed up as many names for body fat as Starbucks has for coffee. Even as otherwise-sensible, well-adjusted adults, many of us spend a huge amount of time dwelling on our double chins, chubby ankles, or flabby arms. We're both fixated and repulsed: We hate our fat, but we can't stop thinking about it.

Well, stop obsessing about your love handles for a minute and ruminate on this: Your fat doesn't just sit there, globlike and idle. Fat is actually a great big gland, churning out hormones and other chemical substances that are essential to many bodily functions. So it's not always bad news. Depending on where it's located, fat may actually protect you from developing heart disease, high blood pressure, or diabetes. But not all fat is created equal. This special report will help you distinguish good fat from the bad, and help you eliminate the latter.

Fat Fundamentals

Basically, fat is stored energy. When you eat, your body transforms carbohydrates, protein, and dietary fat into fatty acids (chains of molecules that are the building blocks of body fat), glucose (blood sugar), or amino acids. These provide energy that you either burn right away or pack up for later. Without body fat, you'd have to eat all the time just to keep your body functioning—your heart beating, your eyes moving across the page, and your hand traveling to your mouth to sip your latte. Fat that isn't used right away gets stored in cells. If you looked at one of them under a microscope, you'd see standard cell equipment—a nucleus, mitochondria, that sort of thing—dwarfed by a big fat droplet that makes up about 85 percent of the cell's volume. Fat cells typically start at five-millionths of a meter in diameter, too tiny to be seen by the naked eye. But they're elastic: Each one can increase by 100 times in volume, to—if you keep stuffing pizza down your throat—about the size of the period at the end of this sentence. For a cell, that's positively ginormous.

For years researchers thought that fat cells were kind of like height: You kept adding to them until you passed puberty, then stopped. But a study published in the *American Journal of Physiology: Endocrinology and Metabolism* found that people actually create new fat cells throughout their adult lives. When a fat cell is full to bursting (i.e., period-size), it sends a chemical signal to surrounding tissue to create new ones. While an average nonoverweight adult has roughly 30 to 40 billion fat cells, someone who's very obese might have as many as 100 billion. And once you've got a fat cell, there's no way to get rid of it, even by losing weight, unless you surgically remove it with liposuction.

In addition to serving as ingenious soft-sided storage bins for our body's energy, fat protects us by providing a layer of insulation that keeps us warm. And it's important to the survival of our species: If a woman's body fat drops below about 18 percent, she stops menstruating and can't reproduce. Nature decides she isn't a good candidate for nourishing an infant. Most important, fat is insurance against starvation. Imagine that Kate Hudson and her chunky cousin (okay, we're not sure she has one) are stranded on a desert island with only water to drink. Kate, assuming she weighs 120 pounds and has 20 percent body fat, could live for 65 days on her fat stores. Her cousin, at 150 pounds and with 30 percent body fat, could last for 105 days—significantly increasing her chances of rescue. What if the two

HOT TIP #50

Bookmark this. Users of an online weight-loss program dropped between 11 and 16 pounds when they were sent e-mail encouragements, compared with just a 6-pound drop among the unprodded, says a study in the *Archives of Internal Medicine*. Sign up for weekly tips at womenshealth.com tried to swim to safety? The heftier gal wins again. That's because fat floats; muscle, which is heavier, doesn't.

Fat doesn't just keep us safe and warm (and above water). It's a busy endocrine factory, secreting substances that play a role in everything from regulating weight to constricting blood vessels. It was the discovery of the hormone leptin in 1994 that woke researchers up to fat's active side. Fat produces leptin, which then travels to the hypothalamus, the part of the brain that controls appetite. There it binds to receptors that send messages signaling that the body is full.

HOT TIP #51

Outrun hunger. Tame cravings with exercise. A British study found that after 58 people worked out every day for 12 weeks, they rated identical breakfasts as 24 percent more filling than they had at the start of the trial. Excercise may raise levels of hormones that affect fullness, says study author Neil King, PhD.

All that said (you knew this was coming), fat does have its downsides. In the past decade, scientists have uncovered more than 100 biochemical substances called adipokines that are created by our fat. Many cause inflammation in tissues and blood vessels, which can raise the risk of heart attack and stroke. Others increase blood pressure or cause clots. Several make our bodies resistant to the effects of insulin, which is what helps move glucose out of the bloodstream and into tissues and organs, where it can be used immediately or stored for energy. About the only bright spot among the adipokines is a hormone called adiponectin, which actually improves the body's response to insulin and reduces the clogging effects of fat on arteries. Unlike the other adipokines, however, you actually make less of this hormone as you get fatter, though no one knows why for sure.

Some fat—specifically, the fat that clusters around our internal organs—also secretes a form of estrogen in both women and men.

(The fat in hips and thighs doesn't.) That can be good and bad. If you're an overweight woman who hasn't yet hit menopause, the extra estrogen may reduce your risk of osteoporosis. On the flip side, it may increase your risk of breast cancer. Although researchers don't know a whole lot about the connection between fat and breast cancer, they suspect that the proximity of visceral fat to a woman's breasts might account for the increased risk. But the relationship between fat and estrogen is even more involved than that. Ovaries produce more estrogen than fat does. When you reach

Decode Any Food Label In Four Easy Steps

Use this simple checklist to outwit the food marketers and find the healthiest products on the shelf. Start with step one, and eliminate products from there.

1. NIX UNHEALTHY FATS: If a product contains partially hydrogenated or interesterified oils, you're eating trans fats, which have been linked to memory impairment, diabetes, and obesity. The words "stearate-rich" mean essentially the same thing.

2. LIMIT SUGARS: Always choose the food with the least amount of sugar. If a product has more than 8 grams, put it back.

3. CHOOSE FIBER: The more, the better, as fiber slows digestion and helps prevent the spikes in blood sugar that lead to obesity and insulin resistance. But buyer beware: Sneaky manufacturers often add isolated fibers such as inulin and maltodextrin to foods so that they can make fiber claims on their packaging, but these are no substitute for whole grains.

4. COUNT INGREDIENTS: Choose the item that is closest to having a list of one.

menopause and the estrogen produced by your ovaries gradually tapers off, a funny thing happens to your fat distribution: It migrates from your hips and thighs to your waist. Researchers think that the lack of estrogen at menopause may play a role in driving fat northward.

Location, Location, Location

Right about now you're thinking, "Okay, how much of this stuff do I have to worry about?" The body of a nonoverweight woman in her twenties or thirties is about 20 to 25 percent fat. By the time she reaches her fifties or sixties, that number will increase to about 28 to 33 percent. "Females are organized to store fat more efficiently than men," says Susan Fried, PhD, an obesity researcher at the University of Maryland School of Medicine. Women pack it away in bigger fat cells and release it very begrudgingly, thanks to higher levels of something called lipoprotein lipase. This enzyme controls the ability of fat cells to grab onto and store away the fat that's circulating in your blood after a meal. No matter how your fat is distributed, though, about 80 percent of it is deposited in squishy pads just beneath the skin of your thighs, butt, stomach, and chest, with smaller pouches in your arms and lower legs. While you may be willing to wager that all of your body fat has made a home on your rear end, it's actually packed around your organs, too, and inside your muscles, like marbling on a steak.

HOT TIP #52

Brew better health. Because of their high yeast content, wheat beers can actually help stabilize blood sugar and may even speed weight loss.

Where your fat is concentrated can make a big difference to your health. Women are more likely to carry fat in their hips, thighs, and buttocks. Researchers are still trying to figure out why precisely this is, but let's face it: You don't need a scientific study for proof. Just look down. But what you probably don't realize is that people who haul around a caboose—a.k.a. "pear-shaped," in popular fruit lingo—have higher HDL (good) cholesterol and lower triglycerides and insulin, putting them at a lower risk for heart disease, high blood pressure, and diabetes. Turns out our hips and thighs provide a roomy storage area for fatty acids to collect instead of circulating through our bloodstream, where they could turn into potentially damaging unstable molecules called free radicals.

For reasons researchers don't yet know, men are much more likely than women to store fat in their midsections, though plenty of women have this "apple shape" as well. We're not talking about that loose flab that makes you rethink leaving the house in your low-rise jeans. That just-below-the-skin, or subcutaneous, fat isn't the most dangerous kind. It's the visceral fat, packed around your liver, heart, and other organs, that poses the biggest health risk. It can clog your arteries and drain right into your liver, where it can impair the organ's vital functions, like converting food into nutrients and removing harmful substances (remember last night's lychee martinis?) from your system. People who have more visceral fat are at higher risk for heart disease, cancer, and diabetes. In fact, many studies have found that waist circumference rather than body mass index (BMI) is the more important factor in determining a person's risk for disease. The good news is that if you lose weight, you'll lose visceral fat more quickly than the kind around your hips and thighs, because it's more easily broken down.

> **HOT TIP #53**
>
> **Trade pounds for dollars.** The average American woman weighs 164 pounds. One study found that being 30 pounds under that average correlates with earning $10,719 more a year.

Your Metabolism under Attack

Now, here's what all this means to you: If your belly is bulging with visceral fat, it's likely that you have the beginnings of something called metabolic syndrome. Metabolic syndrome is a condition in which a woman is inflicted with a cluster of heart-disease risk factors—specifically, a 35-inch (or greater) waist; high triglycerides (the fat in your blood); insulin resisitance or glucose intolerance; and high blood pressure, according to the American Heart Association. This combination increases the likelihood you'll develop diabetes by 500 percent, have a heart attack by 300 percent, and die of a heart attack by 200 percent. (And if you become diabetic, there's an 80 percent chance you'll die of heart disease.)

> **HOT TIP #54**
>
> **Lift weights, eat some nachos.**
> Sometimes—like during an office party —you gotta eat junk. But if you work out beforehand, your muscles will sponge up large amounts of carbs, preventing fat storage.

So how do you know whether your belly houses dangerous levels of visceral fat or the less-dangerous subcutaneous kind? The first step is taking that waist measurement. If it's more than 35 inches, your immediate plan of action—besides a new diet and exercise regimen—should be a visit to the doctor. There, you'll want to request a full metabolic profile. If you have an increasing waistline and any two of the aforementioned requirements for metabolic syndrome, you most assuredly have high amounts of visceral fat. Metabolic syndrome is more common than you think: Recent estimates suggest that it affects 16 percent of women over 20, 37 percent of women between 40 and 59, and 54 percent of women over 60.

Unlike subcutaneous fat, visceral fat can't be liposuctioned away. But it's also easier to target by less-invasive means. Some easy strategies:

How Stress Makes You Fat (In 4 Steps)

1. Stressor

As soon as the stressor hits—an unexpected bill, a mean comment— your glands spring into action.

HYPOTHALAMUS: Responds to stress by secreting corticotrophin-releasing hormone (CRH), which travels to the pituitary gland.

PITUITARY GLAND: Reacts to the CRH by releasing adrenocorticotrophic hormone (ACTH).

ADRENAL GLANDS: Respond to the ACTH by flooding the bloodstream with two stress hormones, epinephrine (a.k.a. adrenaline) and cortisol.

2. Adrenaline

Adrenaline switches on the body's fight-or-flight response:
- Heart rate and pulse quicken to send extra blood to the muscles and organs.
- Bronchial tubes dilate to accept extra oxygen to feed the brain and keep us alert.
- Blood vessels constrict to stem bleeding in case of an injury.

3. Cortisol (your friend)

Cortisol and adrenaline release fat and sugar (glucose) into the bloodstream for use as energy in an emergency. That works perfectly during short-term stress, such as when you need to fend off the angry rottweiler chasing your bike.

4. Cortisol (your enemy)

Cortisol can also signal your cells to store as much fat as possible and inhibit the body from burning it as energy. This occurs because of long-term stress, such as a lunatic boss, a difficult landlord, or a small child who unleashes regular epic tantrums. Chronically elevated cortisol disrupts the body's metabolic control systems: Muscle breaks down, blood sugar rises, appetite increases, and you get fat! What's worse, the fat tends to accumulate in the abdominal region and on the artery walls, because visceral fat has more cortisol receptors than does fat located just under the skin.

GO TO BED EARLIER. A study in Finland looked at sets of identical twins and discovered that of each set of siblings, the twin who slept less and was under more stress had more visceral fat.

BUT HAVE JUST ONE DRINK FIRST. In a study at the State University of New York at Buffalo, the people with the most visceral fat drank only once or twice every 2 weeks but consumed more than four drinks each time. Those with the least visceral fat, on the other hand, drank small amounts of alcohol every day, usually about one drink.

TAKE A WALK. Research shows that the body prefers to use visceral fat for energy, says Robert Ross, PhD, an exercise physiologist at Queen's University in Canada who's been studying the effects of lifestyle on visceral fat for 18 years. In a study published in the journal *Obesity Research*, Ross and his team asked obese women to walk briskly or jog lightly every day for 3 months while eating enough to maintain their weight. The result: They reduced their visceral fat by 18 percent.

GO HARD. Mild exercise whacks away at visceral fat, but strenuous activity has an even greater effect. Canadian researchers found that losing just 11 percent of your body weight can result in a 42 percent reduction in visceral fat; thus, someone who weighs 205 pounds can cut her visceral fat nearly in half by losing 23 pounds. The best weight-loss plan: cardio and strength training, each performed three times a week. Korean scientists found this formula to result in 4 more pounds of weight loss, and 11 percent more visceral fat loss, than cardio alone. (You'll find a plan that works exactly that magic when you read about the *Women's Health* Fast-Track Tone-Up Plan in Chapter 9.)

But keep in mind that the bulge

HOT TIP #55

Turn it up. People could complete 10 additional reps when they listened to their favorite music while exercising, according to a College of Charleston study around your middle isn't entirely your fault to begin with. The American food landscape, with the help of modern "food science," is conspiring to add to that repository of visceral fat. At every rest stop, gas station, airport, mall, and even at the gym, we are surrounded by food that isn't really food at all—it's mostly just varying arrangements of corn and soy mixed with sugar, all of which leads to weight gain if consumed in excess. And, boy do we consume it in excess . . .

Children of the Corn (and Soy)

Practically every packaged food product on the shelves at your local grocery store is made from corn or soy. When researchers from the University of Hawaii analyzed 480 servings of food (hamburgers, chicken sandwiches, and fries) from some of the most popular chain restaurants in the United States (McDonald's, Burger King, and Wendy's), they found that out of the 480 samples, only 12 burgers bought at a Burger King on the West Coast did not show traces of corn. Corn was present in the fat in the fries and in all chicken samples. And they didn't even bother to test the soft drinks, which are basically high-fructose corn syrup (HFCS) and food coloring, or the buns, which are sweetened with HFCS and chock full of soy.

> **HOT TIP #56**
>
> **Maximize minerals.** The bad breath might be worth it: Cooked onions and garlic help your body absorb more of certain key minerals such as iron and zinc from grains, according to a study in the *Journal of Agricultural and Food Chemistry*.

The problem with all that corn and soy is that it means we're eating too much of omega-6 fatty acids—fats that come from seeds like corn kernels and soybeans. (Heart- and brain-healthy omega-3 fatty acids, on the other hand, come from things like seafood, leafy vegetables, and nuts.) And a disproportionately high level of omega-6 fatty acids—a family of fatty acids that compete with omega-3s for space in our cell membranes—promotes chronic inflammation, which leads to heart disease, cancer, Alzheimer's, and depression. Now, we need omega-6s in our diet. They're essential for heart and brain function. But thanks to corn and soy, our foodscape has an omega-6 to omega-3 ratio of about 20:1. Ideally, that ratio should be 1:1.

How did this ratio get so out of whack? Just check the label of any packaged food in your pantry, for starters. If a product contains "polyunsaturated fat," that's usually synonymous with omega-6 fatty acids. So are "high-fructose corn syrup" and "soy protein isolates." In fact, omega-6s have worked their way into virtually all the 45,000 products at your local grocery.

> **HOT TIP #57**
>
> **Go to Rio.** Just four Brazil nuts provide you with 100 percent of your RDA of selenium, a natural anxiety fighter.

And recent research indicates that an out-of-balance omega-6 to omega-3 ratio leads to adipogenesis, or the creation of fat cells! In one study in the *British Journal of Nutrition*, mice fed a ratio of 6:1 omega-6s to omega-3s gained significantly more fat than mice fed a 1:1.2 ratio. Another study in the journal *Progress in Lipid Research* determined that consuming more omega-6s than omega-3s leads to an increased risk of fat development.

The consequences of this can be seen across the country, where 64 percent of American women are overweight and 35 percent are now considered obese. The consumption of HFCS alone, created by chemically altering cornmeal, has been linked to hormonal patterns that promote weight gain. Which is why, even if you've been dieting and exercising, you might not see the results you want.

Target Visceral Fat with This Belly-Busting Workout

Here's how to flatten your gut in less than 30 minutes, three times a week:

1. Weight workout

Choose four upper-body exercises, two lower-body exercises, and two core (abs and lower back) exercises. Do them as a circuit—performing one after the other with no rest in between—but arrange them so that you alternate upper-body exercises with those for your lower body and core. Resting and working your muscles in this way will allow you to work harder in less time, says Jean-Paul Francoeur, the owner of JP Fitness, a health club in Little Rock, Arkansas. Try this circuit: bench press, squat, seated row, stepup, pushup, situp, shoulder press, and back extension. Complete two circuits, resting 2 minutes between them, and do 10 to 15 repetitions of each exercise.

TIME: 18 minutes

2. Cardio workout

Use this interval method. Start out at an easy pace for 90 seconds (about 40 percent of your best effort). Then increase your speed to the fastest pace you can maintain for 30 seconds (about 95 percent of your maximum). That's one interval. Repeat five times, for a total of six intervals. It's short but intense, so it'll save you time. And unlike traditional steady-state aerobic exercise, it'll keep your body burning fat at a higher rate for hours after you're finished. You can perform it on the road or treadmill, but if you're packing more than an extra 20 pounds, opt for an exercise bike to reduce the stress on your knees.

TIME: 12 minutes

TOTAL: 30 minutes

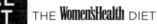
Now, your goal is not to get rid of omega-6s completely, because they are essential to good health. But eating fewer packaged goods and more high-nutrition foods—and focusing on the FAST & LEAN list in Chapter 7—will help bring your intake to more natural levels.

The Unusual Suspects

Food manufacturers sneaking cheap corn and soy into everything from the hamburger bun to the hamburger itself is just one force you have to fight against. Here's a look at how stress, chemicals, hidden sugars, lack of sleep, and crafty food marketing are battling against your weight loss efforts every day:

STRESS: Whether you're fending off a toddler meltdown, an angry client, or a disgruntled spouse, your body's response to stress is the same: Your hypothalamus floods your blood with hormones to frighten you into action. Cortisol and epinephrine are your body's alarm-system hormones; they make your heart beat faster and dilate your bronchial tubes so they can feed oxygen to your brain and keep you alert. They also release fat and glucose into your bloodstream to provide emergency energy. But too much stress keeps your cortisol levels consistently elevated, which disrupts your metabolic system. This, in turn, signals your cells to store as much fat as possible. Worse, the fat tends to accumulate in your belly as dangerous visceral fat, which resides behind your abdominal muscles and has more cortisol receptors than other fat does. (For a blow-by-blow on this chemical process, see "How Stress Makes You Fat," on page 73.)

> **HOT TIP #58**
>
> **Don't patrol the border.** The average margarita has 3 times as many calories as a Cosmopolitan and 4½ times as many as a glass of wine.

FIGHT BACK: To defend yourself against stress-induced weight gain, make a habit of exercising 3 days a week. Doing so helps regulate your cortisol levels, say researchers at Ohio State University. Also, try to eat organic foods as much as possible, in order to steer clear of the common pesticide atrazine. A National Health and Environmental Effects Research Laboratory study showed that atrazine produced extreme increases in stress-hormone levels in rats. In fact, the stress reaction was similar to that seen when the animals were restrained against their will, the study noted.

ENDOCRINE-DISRUPTING CHEMICALS: There's a new threat to your belly—a class of natural and synthetic compounds known as endocrine disrupting chemicals (EDCs), or, as researchers have begun to call them, obesogens. Obesogens are chemicals that disrupt the function of our endocrine systems, leading to weight gain and many of the diseases that curse the American populace. Because high school biology was probably a while back, here's a quick refresher: The endocrine system is made up of all the glands and cells that produce the hormones that regulate our bodies. Growth and development, sexual function, reproductive processes, mood, sleep, hunger, stress, metabolism, and the way our bodies use food—it's all controlled by hormones. But your endocrine system is a finely tuned instrument that can easily be thrown off kilter. "Obesogens are thought to act by hijacking the regulatory systems that control body weight," says Frederick vom Saal, PhD, curators' professor of biological sciences at the University of Missouri. That's why endocrine disruptors are so good at making us fat,

> **HOT TIP #59**
>
> **Eat a better butter.** Almond butter has more calcium and magnesium, 60 percent more healthy fat, and three times as much vitamin E as peanut butter.

and that's why diet advice doesn't always work, because even strictly following the smartest traditional advice won't lower your obesogen exposure. See, an apple a day may have kept the doctor away 250 years ago, when Benjamin Franklin included the phrase in his almanac. But if that apple comes loaded with obesity-promoting chemicals—nine of the 10 most commonly used pesticides are obesogens, and apples are one of the most pesticide-laden foods out there—then Ben's advice is way out-of-date.

HOT TIP #60

Stand up for your health.
Your core works 20 percent harder when performing a standing cable chest press than during a standard barbell bench press.

FIGHT BACK: Obesogens enter our bodies from a wide variety of sources—from natural hormones found in soy products, from artificial hormones fed to our animals, from plastic pollutants in some food packaging, from chemicals added to processed foods, and from pesticides sprayed on our produce. See "Your Guide to Avoiding Endocrine-Disrupting, Fat-Inducing Chemicals" (on page 84) for details on how to cleanse your body of these nasty fat-promoting invaders.

HIDDEN SUGARS: Eat a little sugar and you end up craving more, which means more calories and a bigger waist. That's because sugar is addictive, seriously addictive. A group of Princeton researchers found that eating sugar triggers the release of opioids, neurotransmitters that activate the brain's pleasure receptors. Addictive drugs, including morphine, target the same opioid receptors. That's right, sugar activates the same pathways that are stimulated by drugs such as heroin and morphine. Which explains why we eat so much of it. According to a USDA survey, the average American eats about 20 teaspoons of added sugar daily, or 317 empty calories.

Eight-two percent of that added sugar is from soda, baked goods, breakfast cereals, candy, and fruit drinks. But sugar shows up in so many products and under so many different names that you may not even know you're eating it. Look for these aliases: maltose, sorghum, sorbitol, dextrose, lactose, fructose, high fructose corn syrup, and glucose. And then there are the healthy-sounding versions: barley malt, brown rice sugar, fruit juice, honey, molasses, and organic cane juice.

FIGHT BACK: All sugars spike insulin levels and affect the body in the same way. A good rule is to skip any product that lists sugar as one of its first four ingredients. And do your best to avoid fructose. New research from the University of California, San Francisco (UCSF), indicates that fructose (our greatest source of fructose is high-fructose corn syrup, with an average daily consumption of 12 teaspoons) can trick your brain into craving more food, even when you're full. Preliminary research indicates that fructose may play a role in disrupting our endocrine systems by interfering with our ability to process leptin, the hormone that tells us when we're full, says Robert Lustig, MD, a pediatric endocrinologist at UCSF. But it's not just high-fructose corn syrup and table syrup that you need to avoid; fruit juice can be as bad as soda. In fact, 100 percent fruit juice has 1.8 grams of fructose per ounce, while soda has 1.7 grams per ounce.

> **HOT TIP #61**
>
> **Shed water weight.** Got water-retention woes? Skip salt-laden foods (that includes all takeout) for potassium power-houses like avocados and bananas, which will help get rid of the extra fluid.

SLEEPLESSNESS: A sleep schedule is vital to any weight-loss plan. Too much or too little shut-eye can add extra pounds. In a new study, Canadian scientists revealed that sleeping for 5 to 6 hours a night makes you 69 percent more likely to pack on pounds than if you log 8 hours. What's just as surprising is that snoozing for 9 to 10 hours also increases your risk of becoming overweight by 38 percent. "Lack of sleep releases hormones that stimulate your appetite," says study author Jean-Philippe Chaput, MSc. "But oversleeping means you'll burn less energy in a day, since you aren't as active." Plus, an Australian study found that dozing late on weekends leaves you more tired Monday and Tuesday, compared with sticking to your workday wake-up time. People with sleep deficits tend to eat more (and use less energy) because they're tired, according to Wake Forest University researchers, while those who sleep longer than 8 hours a night may be less active.

FIGHT BACK: Make sure you have good melatonin rhythm. When the sun goes down, your pineal gland switches on like clockwork to secrete melatonin, a hormone that helps you fall asleep and regulates your circadian rhythm. It lowers your core body temperature, which, if too high, promotes wakefulness. Production of melatonin peaks in the middle of the night, and the process can be disrupted by even very low levels of artificial light. Darkness is the key to good melatonin rhythm. Buy heavy curtains, cover your alarm clock, and turn off gadgets. Make it dark enough that you can't see your hand. If you go to the bathroom and turn on that bright light, you'll lower melatonin almost immediately. So use a red night-light (or heat lamp) in your bathroom, because red light has less effect on melatonin than white or blue light.

> **HOT TIP #62**
>
> **Whip your shake.** You can boost the appetite-suppressing effect of a whey shake by whipping it to a froth. Penn State researchers found that people who drank more aerated shakes ate 12 percent less food at their next meal. Scientists speculate that the froth made men think they were drinking more.

SNEAKY SUPERMARKET TRICKS: Food manufacturers think you're stupid. And their marketing strategies rely on it. For instance, the makers of Swedish Fish, Mike and Ike, and Good & Plenty may be hoping you'll equate the "fat-free" label they have plastered on their candy boxes with "healthy" or "nonfattening" so you'll forget about all the sugar their products contain. It's a distraction device: Food companies advertise what they want you to notice—and the candy aisle is just the start. They can also get away with marking their calorie counts in a misleading way—for example, declaring that a small bottle of juice to be 2½ servings when clearly you're meant to drink the whole thing. Many packaged food offenders are obvious— you already know that the double-cheese-and-pepperoni calzones are a health hazard—but a lot of the worst products are double agents. They pose as healthy choices, labeled with such comforting words as "fortified," "lite," "all-natural," and even "multigrain." But you'd be surprised to discover how meaningless these words are in reality.

FIGHT BACK: Think of the grocery store as a battleground and the edges of the store—where produce, dairy, and meat are sold—as your green zone. Stay there and make only strategic, solo incursions into the middle aisles to snag beans and whole-grain cereals. But be aware: A label that says, "made with whole grain" doesn't necessarily mean a healthy food. Pick up a box of Franken Berry and you'll see what we mean. A product needs to be made of only 51 percent whole-grain flour in order to carry this label. To make sure you're getting a truly whole-grain product, check that the word "whole" is next to every flour listed. And know that the newest marketing ploy, describing foods as "all-natural," has no specific government standards and there's no legislation for it. Just about anything can be called all-natural.

Your Guide to Avoiding Endocrine-Disrupting, Fat-Inducing Chemicals

Our foods, even foods we consider "health" or "diet" foods, are loaded with endocrine-disrupting chemicals that prime your body for fat storage. Here's what you need to do to avoid them.

KNOW WHEN TO GO ORGANIC. The average American is exposed to 10 to 13 different pesticides through food, beverages, and drinking water every day, and 9 of the 10 most common pesticdes are endocrine-disrupting chemicals, or EDCs—chemicals that hijack metabolism and cause you to store fat. Researchers have even coined a term to explain their threat: they call them "obesogens." But according to a recent study in the journal *Environmental Health Perspectives*, eating an organic diet for just 5 days can reduce circulating pesticide EDCs to non-detectable or near-nondetectable levels. Of course, organic foods can be expen-sive. But you don't have to be 100 percent organic—many foods have such low levels of pesticides that buying organic just isn't worth it. The Environmental Working Group (EWG) calculated that you can reduce your pesticide exposure by nearly 80 percent simply by choosing organic for the 12 fruits and vegetables shown in their tests to contain the highest levels of pesticides: celery, peaches, strawberries, apples, blueberries (domestic), nectarines, sweet bell peppers, spinach, kale/collard greens, cherries, potatoes, and grapes (imported). As a general rule of thumb, if you can eat it without peeling it, go organic.

DON'T EAT PLASTIC. You're probably think-ing, "Well, I don't gen-erally eat plastic." Ah, but you do. Chances are that you're among the 93 percent of Americans with detectable levels of bisphenol-A (BPA) in their bodies and that you're also among the 75 percent of Ameri-cans with detectable levels of phthalates. Both are synthetic chemicals that mimic estrogen—essentially, artificial female hor-mones—and they leach into our foods from plastic or alumi-num food packaging. These plastic-based chemicals trick our bodies into storing fat and not building or retaining muscle. Decreasing your exposure to plastic-

based obesogens will maximize your chances both of losing unwanted flab and of building lean muscle mass. Here's how:
1. Never heat food in plastic containers or put plastic items in the dishwasher, which can increase the amount of BPA they release. BPA leaches from polycarbonate sports bottles 55 times faster when exposed to boiling liquids as opposed to cold ones, according to a study in the journal *Toxicology Letters*.
2. Avoid buying fatty foods like meats that are packaged in plastic wrap, because EDCs are stored in fatty tissue. The plastic wrap used at the supermarket is mostly PVC, whereas the plastic wrap you buy to wrap things at home is increasingly made from more benign polyethylene.
3. Cut down on canned goods; choose food like tuna in a pouch instead of a can.

GO LEAN. Whenever possible, choose pasture-raised meats, which, studies show, have less fat than their confined, grain-fed counterparts and none of the weight-promoting hormones. Plus, grass-fed beef contains 60 percent more omega-3s, 200 percent more vitamin E, and two to three times more conjugated linoleic acid (CLA, a nutrient that helps ward off heart disease, cancer, and diabetes and can help you lose weight, according to a study in the *American Journal of Clinical Nutrition*) than conventionally raised beef. And select sustainable lean fish with low levels of toxins like mercury and PCBs. A study in the journal *Occupational and Environmental Medicine* found that even though the pesticide DDT was banned in 1973, the chemical and its breakdown product, DDE, can still be found today in fatty fish. Bigger fish eat smaller fish and so carry a much higher toxic load. Avoid ahi or bigeye tuna, tilefish, swordfish, shark, and marlin. Focus on smaller fish like anchovies, and mackerel and wild-caught Alaskan salmon. Choose farmed rainbow trout, farmed mussels, scallops (bay, farmed), Pacific halibut, tuna, and mahimahi. When you cook fish, broil, grill, or bake it instead of pan-frying—this will allow contaminants from the fatty portions of fish to drain out.

FILTER YOUR WATER. The best way to eliminate EDCs from your tap water is an activated carbon water filter. Available for faucets and pitchers and as under-the-sink units, these filters remove most pesticides and industrial pollutants. Check the label to make sure the filter meets the National Science Foundation/American National Standards Institute's standard 53, indicating that it treats water for both health and aesthetic concerns.

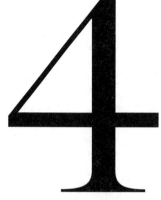

WHY THE SMARTEST DIET IS NO DIET AT ALL

How to turn fat into muscle without giving up anything, ever.

By this stage in our story, you've already learned a thing or two about fitness, nutrition, and weight loss. You've done simple exercises to help you measure your personal fitness level, and you've picked up plenty of cool tips on looking and feeling your best. Now you're ready to head into a bold new future—with a bold new body. But before we charge forward, we have one more subject to cover. Answer this question correctly, and you'll be ready to move on to our next round.

You are most likely headed for a future of obesity if . . .

A) The closest you get to regular exercise is reaching for another handful of Cheetos.

B) The street address on your driver's license is "Kirstie Alley."

C) You think the term "fruit-and-nut bar" refers to where you met your ex.

D) You are currently, right now, at this very moment, on a diet.

And the answer is: D!

It seems counterintuitive, but studies have shown time and again that the biggest predictor of becoming overweight in the future is whether you're on a diet RIGHT NOW. Indeed, almost every diet plan out there is designed to make you gain pounds in the long term.

Wow. Really? WTF?

(And also, why did I just shell out big bucks for this *Women's Health Diet* book when I could have put the money toward that sweet new Marc Jacobs tote?)

Well, first off, we said that almost every diet plan out there will make you gain flab. The *Women's Health* Nutrition System is a different animal entirely. But before we explain how, let us tell you what's wrong with the others.

The Trouble with Traditional Diets

There are tens of thousands of diet plans out there, touted by doctors, by celebrities, by athletes—all sorts of schemes, some sensible and most pretty crazy. And every single one of them has one thing in common: They will all work, until they don't.

You see, every diet works to a certain degree, because every diet you go on forces you to pay attention to the food you eat, and that alone helps cut down on your calorie intake. Who cares if some of those schemes sound a little wacky—grapefruit diets, cabbage soup diets, cottage cheese diets, mayonnaise-and-Slim-Jim diets? (Okay, we made that last one up.) And who cares if the natural act of eating becomes an exercise in trigonometry as you try to calculate your calorie intake and phases and "pods" and ratios and points and all the other bizarre mathematical formulas out there? The good news for the nearly 76 million Americans who are on a diet of some kind at this very moment is that, in the short term, every single of them will work.

And the bad news? In the long term, say UCLA researchers, two-thirds of people who lose weight on a diet plan end up weighing more than when they started! Heck, diets are the Florida condo markets of health and fitness.

So how do you know whether a diet is destined to fail? The same way you can tell whether your car is about to die or a relationship is getting stale: You heed the warning signs. Here, then, is the 3-Point *Women's Health* Diet Diagnostic.

> **HOT TIP #63**
>
> **Get a milk mustache.** Consuming 1,800 milligrams of calcium a day could block the absorption of about 80 calories, according to a University of Tennessee study. Jump-start your intake by filling your coffee mug with milk, drinking it down to the level you want in your coffee, then pouring in the java. That's 300 milligrams!

TROUBLE SIGN #1: You have to eliminate an entire food group. When a diet calls itself "low fat" or "low carb" or involves "cleansing" your body with shakes and smoothies, that's not weight loss magic; that's calorie restriction. A recent study in the *New England Journal of Medicine* found that, regardless of the type of diet you choose—whether it bans carbs or fats or sodium or meat or dairy or, heck, frittatas and fruitcakes—it will lead to weight loss, because banning a particular food group will automatically create a calorie deficit. This finding is echoed in other recent studies published in the journals *Diabetes Care*, the *American Journal of Clinical Nutrition*, and *The Archives of Internal Medicine*. But the thing about calorie restriction is that it's not sustainable, it can actually be harmful (especially if you're concerned about forming and maintaining lean muscle), and it leads to weight gain down the road. Recently, scientists reporting in the journal *Psychosomatic Medicine* investigated how the body reacts when you (a) monitor your caloric intake or (b) restrict your caloric intake. They found that restricting calories increases circulating levels of the stress hormone cortisol (which tells your body trouble's brewing and basically forces you to store calories as flab to prepare for hard times) and even just monitoring calories increases perceived stress. They concluded that "dieting, or the restriction of caloric intake, is ineffective because it increases chronic psychological stress and cortisol production, two factors that are known to cause weight gain." The study's authors added that dieting in general seems to be harmful to your psychological as well as physical well-being. (That's why the *Women's Health* Diet is all about eating more, not eating less.)

> **HOT TIP #64**
>
> **Skip the sodas.** Chugging two or more sodas a week could raise your risk of pancreatic cancer by 87 percent according to a study published in *Cancer Epidemiology, Biomarkers & Prevention.*

TROUBLE SIGN #2: You have to follow a formula, algorithm, or point-tallying system to figure out what to eat. Cognitive scientists from Indiana University and the Max Planck Institute for Human Development, in Berlin, recently discovered that the more complex a diet appears to be, the more likely you are to quit it. The researchers compared the results of women following the Weight Watchers point system and women following a simple diet that recommended specific foods and meals. They found that simply perceiving that your diet plan is complex (regardless of how simple it actually might be) makes it 54 percent more likely that you will prematurely give up said diet. (That's why we made the *Women's Health* Diet so simple—all you need to do is eyeball your portions as outlined later, so you won't have to tax your brain to follow it.)

TROUBLE SIGN #3: You're told that if you base your diet around one single nutrient or food, you'll lose weight. You've seen them advertised: the apple diet, the apple cider vinegar diet, the pineapple diet (and those are just a few that include the word "apple"!) These strange fad diets are two things: (1) calorie restriction in disguise and (2) deprivation diets that don't let you enjoy the full bounty of nutrition that nature has to offer. For both of these reasons, diets like these are unsustainable and will ultimately lead to rebound weight gain. We simply can't exist on a narrow spectrum of food. Our taste buds crave diversity, and for good reason: A varied diet is a healthy diet. So, when we deny ourselves nutrition for the sake of weight loss, our bodies rebel. A study published in the *International Journal of Obesity* found that 91 percent of people starting a diet experienced food cravings; and that figure went even higher as

> **HOT TIP #65**
>
> **Block blisters.**
> For long workouts, spread a little bit of Vaseline on the bottom of your feet and in between your toes. This will keep sweaty feet from blistering.

HOT TIP #66

Ruin your appetite. Consuming a liquid—whether it's two glasses of water or a cup of soup—to begin a meal can fill you up and reduce your total calorie intake by up to 20 percent. Try this: Drink one glass of H$_2$O and have a broth-based soup, such as miso, minestrone, or chicken noodle, as an appetizer.

the calorie restriction continued. And—this is the really creepy part—every time you resist a piece of pie, or a bagel with cream cheese, or whatever your favorite indulgence is, you decrease your chances of being able to say no the next time. That's because the ability to control ourselves wanes after we first exert self-control, according to a new study from Florida State University. The reason? Self-control is fueled by . . . wait for it . . . sugar—glucose, to be exact. So every time you say no to those carbs, you increase your need for the very nutrients they contain. Ouch!

Indeed, most popular diets are just variations on the three themes discussed above. Let's take a tour through some of the top weight-loss plans out there and see whether anything looks familiar.

The Zone Diet

The guiding principle of this particular diet is that high insulin levels contribute to weight gain, and therefore stabilizing insulin leads to weight loss. Okay, sounds reasonable. But to accomplish this goal, every meal has to have a specific ratio of carbs, protein, and fat (40 percent carbs, 30 percent protein, and 30 percent fat). That's the "zone" you need to be in all the time. You eat low-fat proteins at every meal; focus on good fats like the monounsaturated fat in olive oil, almonds, and avocados and the omega-3 fatty acids in fish; limit carb intake to whole grains and some fruits while avoiding juice, beer, and sweets; restrict saturated fat from red meat and egg yolks; and avoid processed foods. Whew. And that's just the basic diet. Foods are grouped into "blocks" based on their protein, fat, and carb content, so that one block of food will deliver the magical 40: 30: 30 ratio. And then you are allotted so many blocks a day depending on how much you exercise.

Now, the Zone gets credit for trying to balance essential nutrients while attempting not to restrict too many foods. But, according to a recent study in the *Journal of the American Medical Association*, the diet has the same effect on insulin levels as all the other popular diets. So basically all that counting of carbs, proteins, and fats and making sure they're proportioned right for each meal does little more than make you hyperaware of the foods you're eating, which can help you cut back on calories and lose weight.

And did you recognize one or more of the dietary trouble signs? Yep, Trouble Sign #2 stands out: This diet is way too complex and therefore is probably unsustainable. To be fair, the Zone does offer prepackaged foods that fit its formula, but they're highly processed and seriously unnatural—in fact, these "food" products were among the many diet aids that were recalled by their manufacturer in 2009 for containing tainted peanut butter. We're here to tell you that the *Women's Health* Diet is a better way.

HOT TIP #67

Hold for muscles. Simply holding barbells or dumbbells strengthens your wrists and forearms by as much as 25 percent and 16 percent, respectively, in 12 weeks, according to a study at Auburn University.

The Atkins Diet

It's a low-carbohydrate, high-fat diet consisting of four phases. Phase 1 eliminates almost all carbohydrates (you're allowed only 20 grams a day—that means no bread, pasta, fruit, vegetables, or juice, just proteins and fats). Phase 2 increases carbohydrate intake to 25 grams a day, and each week thereafter you increase your carb intake by 5 grams, continuing like this until you stop losing weight. Phase 3 is when you decrease your carb intake by 5 grams daily to reinitiate weight loss. Phase 4 is based on the number of grams of carbs you need to maintain your weight. We don't know about you, but aside from needing a cookie every now and again, going without fruits and vegetables—the very foods that study after study say are the key to health and longevity—seems counterproductive.

The diet's emphasis on protein is on the right track—a recent study in the *American Journal of Clinical Nutrition* found that those who get 30 percent of their daily calories from protein feel more satiated than those who eat less protein, leading them to consume 441 fewer calories a day and lose 5 pounds over 2 weeks. But Atkins takes this idea to the extreme. And in reality, it's just camouflaged calorie restriction. Of course you're going to lose weight if you restrict a nutrient group completely! But you're also losing out on a whole spectrum of wonderful tastes, smells, and textures that your body craves. This diet is guilty of all three trouble signs!

Which means it's just not sustainable. Restricting foods will only make you crave them more, and you may end up bingeing instead. The bottom line is that you might lose weight to begin with, but keeping it off is another story. Again, the *Women's Health Diet* is a better, tastier way.

Weight Watchers

Here, every food has a value based on its calorie, fat, and fiber content per serving. Fiber decreases the point value assigned to a particular food, whereas fat and calories increase the point value. Your job is to stay under a certain number of points every day in order to achieve your weight-loss goals. You can choose between a high-carb or a high-protein plan.

The folks at Weight Watchers deserve credit for helping people realize how many calories they're putting into their bodies. And they're really focused on providing social support, an important aspect of weight management. But while monitoring daily calorie intake is a great exercise for those who want to lose weight, ultimately, it is just that—an exercise. Counting calories is not something that you want to do for the rest of your life. Food is meant to be enjoyed, after all. On top of that, the point system can have the unintended effect of slowing your metabolism if, say, you eat all of your points in one meal and then starve yourself for the rest of the day (more on that later). This diet is the poster child for Trouble Sign #2.

THE BOTTOM LINE FOR ALL OF THESE DIETS IS THIS: Gimmicks don't work. No portion ratio or carb restriction or point system is going to help you navigate the food you're confronted with every day. The *Women's Health* Nutrition System takes into account the reality of your environment and offers you a diet—no, a lifestyle—that allows you to eat the foods you crave and helps you shed pounds and keep them off.

5

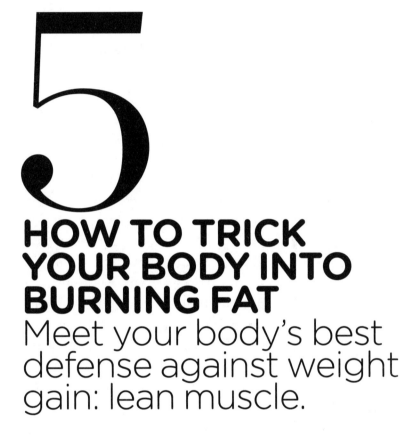

HOW TO TRICK YOUR BODY INTO BURNING FAT

Meet your body's best defense against weight gain: lean muscle.

How would you like to magically burn off about 40 calories in the next 15 minutes, without even breaking a sweat? Want to try? Okay, here's what you do:

Go into the bedroom. Open up the closet.

Look inside. Anything need to go to the dry cleaner? What about that pashmina you spilled New Year's bubbly on? Toss it in the laundry bag. Straighten a few hanging items and refold your sweaters so the inside of your wardrobe doesn't look like you had to flee the paparazzi. Good job. Now have a seat.

Ta-da! You've just smoked 40 or more calories in less time than it takes to put on your makeup, and all you did was neaten up your clothes. Magic, right?

Well, not really. You see, your body is already primed to be a fat-burning machine. All you need to do to start changing your body's shape is tune up that fat furnace and get it revving at maximum efficiency so you're burning even more fat while going about the mundane rituals of life.

> **HOT TIP #69**
>
> **Start slow.** In a study in *Obesity*, women who ranked their workouts the toughest packed on the most pounds over the next 12 months. A negative experience with exercise makes it harder to adopt a long-term workout plan, says study author David Brock, PhD, of the University of Vermont.

This fat-burning magic comes from your metabolism, a word you've probably heard tossed around a lot but maybe don't quite understand. What is metabolism? Simply put, it's all the various chemical reactions that happen inside your body, 24-7, that keep you alive. It's food being turned into energy and that energy being burned off to keep your hair growing, your heart beating, your liver pumping out bile, your lungs transferring oxygen into your bloodstream, and your intestines turning Amstel Light into urine (not that there's a huge leap there). It's the engine room of your individual starship, your never-ending calorie burn. And while you may imagine that the majority of your calories get burned while you're engaged in some strenuous activity like riding a bike, diving into a pool, or getting jiggy with your honey, you're actually burning most of your calories, well, just keeping the lights on.

In fact, think of metabolism as your caloric 401(k) program. It's not going to give you instant gratification, like hitting a slot machine jackpot. It's a long-term strategy, but it's a sure thing: Invest in it and you'll get slow, steady, effective returns that will keep you happy and healthy for years to come.

Now, like any long-term investment, it needs a little maintenance from time to time. In this chapter, we'll show you the smart ways to tweak your metabolism, improving your burn just enough to gain even more over the long haul. (Or to borrow what they say in financial circles, it's time to work less for your calorie burn and have your calorie burn start working for you!) Prepare for a few surprises, starting with . . .

Why Burning Calories in the Gym Is a Waste of Time

Whoa—did we just say what you thought we said? That burning calories in the gym is "a waste of time"? Is this really a *Women's Health* book?

Well, stay with us here. Burning calories in the gym is great—in fact, in Chapter 8, you'll learn about the *Women's Health* Fast-Track Tone-Up Plan, our most effective fat-burning plan ever, designed to burn close to 130 calories off a 140-pound woman in just 15 minutes (that's 500-plus an hour!). But the energy you expend while you're in the gym isn't as simple as those tired old LED readouts on the treadmill might make it seem. See, we all have three "burns" that make up our metabolism:

Burn One

Basal (resting) metabolism: Your basal metabolic rate (BMR) accounts for 60 to 70 percent of your overall metabolism, and surprisingly, it's the number of calories you burn doing nothing at all: lying in bed staring at the ceiling or vegging on the couch watching TV. As we said earlier, it's fueled by your body's inner workings—your heart beating, your lungs breathing, even your cells dividing.

Burn Two

Digestive metabolism, or thermic effect of food (TEF): Simply digesting food—turning carbs into sugar and turning protein into amino acids—typically burns 10 to 15 percent of your daily calories. Digesting protein burns more calories than digesting carbohydrates or fat—about 25 calories for every 100 consumed. Digesting carbohydrates and fat burns about 10 to 15 calories for every 100 consumed. (You'll see why this is important to remember in Chapter 6.)

HOT TIP #70

Seed for the future. Pumpkin seeds are the easiest way to consume more magnesium, which French researchers have linked to longevity.

So pause a moment to think about this: Between 70 and 85 percent of the calories you burn every day come from either eating or just hanging around doing nothing.

So, what about the other 15 to 30 percent?

Burn Three

Exercise and movement metabolism: This part of your metabolism includes both workouts at the gym and other more enjoyable physical activities (we call this exercise-activity thermogenesis, or EAT) along with countless incidental movements throughout the day, like turning the pages of this book and twiddling your thumbs (that's called non-exercise-activity thermogenesis, or NEAT).

So, here's an interesting question: Why is it so hard to lose weight just by exercising? Why are there so many fat people in the gym? The answer is simple. Exercise only targets 15 to 30 percent of your fat burn. Up to 85 percent of the calories you burn in a given day have nothing to do with moving your body!

So, skip the gym, right? Not quite.

Why the Fatter You Get, the Fatter You'll Get

Fat doesn't just show up at your door one day, rent a room, and live alone quietly. Fat loves company. Fat's organizing a cocktail party where nobody ever goes home and everyone hangs out around your midsection. The more fat you open the door to, the harder it will be to stop even more fat from inviting itself in. Here's why:

Your BMR, or resting metabolism—the body system that eats up the majority of your daily calorie burn—is determined by two things: your parents, and the amount of fat versus muscle in your body. And while you can't choose who your parents are (if you could, there would be no children on *The Real Housewives of New Jersey*), you can improve the other part of the equation and turn your resting metabolism up a few notches.

Problem is, fat plays its own role in the metabolic game, and it's literally working to slow down your calorie burn. See, the term "fat and lazy" is pretty accurate from a scientific standpoint. Fat is lazy, on a metabolic level. It barely burns any calories at all. For your body to support a pound of fat, it needs to burn a mere 2 calories a day.

HOT TIP #71

Get juiced for sleep. Cherry juice is a concentrated source of melatonin, an effective sleep aid. Just beware of juice blends with high levels of sugar.

Muscle, on the other hand, is very metabolically active. This is key (and why muscle is your BFF): At rest, 1 pound of muscle burns three times as many calories every day just to sustain itself—and a lot of those calories that muscle burns off come from fat's storage units. That's why fat hates muscle (and why you should love muscle), because muscle is constantly burning fat off.

So fat actually fights back, trying to erode muscle and fit more of its fat friends into your body. The real villain in this internal battle happening right now, in your body, is a nasty character called visceral fat. As you read in our special report "A Matter of Fat" on page 65, visceral fat is the kind that resides behind the abdominal muscles, surrounding your internal organs (viscera). And visceral fat works its mischief by releasing a number of substances, collectively called adipokines. Adipokines include compounds that raise your risk of high blood pressure, diabetes, inflammation, and heart disease. Visceral fat also messes with an important hormone called adiponectin, which regulates metabolism.

HOT TIP #72

Stick it to tartar.
People who chewed sugar-free gum (ones with xylitol, a sugar alcohol) had 33 percent less tartar on their teeth.

The more visceral fat you have, the less adiponectin you have, and the lower your metabolism. So fat literally begets more fat.

A study published in the *Journal of Applied Physiology* showed that those biologically active molecules that are released from visceral fat can actually degrade muscle quality—which, again, leads to more fat. The solution?

More muscle.

After age 25 we all start to lose muscle mass—a fifth of a pound of muscle a year, from ages 25 to 50, and then up to a pound of muscle a year after that—if we don't do anything to stop the decline. And on top of a slumping metabolic rate, loss of muscle strength and mass are empirically linked to declines in the immune system,

How to Burn Off 21 Pounds This Year Without Feeling a Thing

CONSIDER THIS: If you burn 10 additional calories a day, you'll lose a pound a year. So if you could burn off a mere 210 calories a day, you could lose 21 pounds. And you could do that without ever stepping foot in a gym. You just need to tweak your everyday routine.

CASE IN POINT: Incorporate the strategies below into your life and you can effortlessly—burn about 10 percent more calories a day.*

+	+	+	+	+
DO THIS	**DO THIS**	**DO THIS**	**DO THIS**	**DO THIS**
Go for a brisk 20-minute walk	Stand during three 10-minute phone calls	Play vigorously with your kids or pet for 15 minutes	Spend 15 minutes washing the dishes	Take 10 minutes to straighten up one room
—	**—**	**—**	**—**	**—**
NOT THIS	**NOT THIS**	**NOT THIS**	**NOT THIS**	**NOT THIS**
Sit for your entire lunch hour	Put your feet up on your desk	Watch TV before dinner	Head straight to the couch	Go right to bed
=	**=**	**=**	**=**	**=**
49 extra calories burned	33 extra calories burned	82 extra calories burned	27 extra calories burned	21 extra calories burned

TOTAL: 210 calories!

*Based on a 140-pound woman

not to mention weaker bones, stiffer joints, and slumping postures. Muscle mass also plays a central role in the response to stress. And further research is expected to show measurable links between diminished muscle mass and cancer mortality.

Muscle mass has also proved to play a key role in preventing more common but no less deadly conditions such as cardiovascular disease and diabetes. A study of scientific literature published in the journal *Circulation* in 2006 linked the loss of muscle mass to insulin resistance (the main factor in adult-onset, or type 2, diabetes), elevated lipid levels in the blood, and increased body fat, especially visceral fat.

See? It's a war. And if you want to stop the bad guy—visceral fat—you need to call in reinforcements.

Why the Most Important Calories You Can Burn Are the Ones You're Burning Right Now

As you've seen on the previous pages, muscle is your body's defense system against the onslaught of fat. That's why the *Women's Health* Fast-Track Tone-Up Plan is the perfect armament upgrade. It's a simple weight-training regimen with an aerobic edge that will help your body attack fat even while you're at rest. It works in three simple ways for three simple reasons:

First, as we said earlier, a pound of flab burns only 2 calories a day, while the same amount of skeletal muscle burns an estimated 6 calories a day, researchers believe. "Many factors are at play, so call this the best-educated guess," says Jeff Volek, PhD, RD, an exercise and nutrition expert at the University of Connecticut. So the more muscle you have, the more fat you burn, all day every day.

That's why the *Women's Health* Fast-Track Tone-Up Plan focuses on adding lean muscle to your physique.

Second, while muscle burns calories, new muscle burns more calories. That's because the physical work you need to do to build and maintain new muscle can have a dramatic effect on your overall metabolism. Research shows that a single weight-training session can spike your calorie burn for up to 39 hours afterward. (And remember, that's not including the calories you be burned off while you're actually exercising—roughly 8.5 calories a minute, or 508 an hour. Think of those as just a bonus.)

The long-term calorie burn you get through weight-training doesn't just get rid of extra weight. It specifically targets belly fat! In a study conducted by Jeff Volek, overweight people following a reduced-calorie diet were divided into three groups. One group didn't exercise, the second performed aerobic exercise 3 days a week, and the third did both aerobics and weight-training 3 days a week. The results: Each group lost about the same amount of weight—21 pounds on average per person in 12 weeks. But those who lifted weights shed 5 pounds more fat than those who didn't pump iron. The weight they lost was almost pure fat, while the other two groups shed 15 pounds of lard but also 5-plus pounds of muscle. "Think about that," says Volek. "For the same amount of exercise time, with diets being equal, the participants who lifted weights lost almost 40 percent more fat."

> **HOT TIP #73**
>
> **Stagger yourself.** The next time you do pushups, stagger your hands—it'll increase the challenge to your core and shoulder muscles.

And there's a third, even more exciting reason why weight-training is the ultimate fat-fighter: The more muscle you have, the better your body's ability to use the nutrients you eat—and the less likely it is to store your food (even junk food) as fat.

See, your muscles store energy (read: calories) in the form of glycogen. When you exercise, your muscles have to call on that glycogen to perform the work they're being tasked with doing. (When you get that weak-kneed feeling at the end of a treadmill session, that's your leg muscles telling you their glycogen tank is hitting zero.) One of the many advantages to working out is that after you exercise, your fat-storing hormones are dimmed, because your

Burn, Baby, Burn
Calories burned per hour by a 140-pound woman

1. SITTING AT A DESK **114**
2. HAVING SEX **125**
3. PLAYING VOLLEYBALL **254**
4. CANOEING **286**
5. GOLFING **286**
6. KAYAKING **318**
7. HIKING **381**
8. SURFING **400**
9. PLAYING TENNIS **445**
10. DOING BODY-WEIGHT CALISTHENICS IN THE SAND ...... **222 - 508**
11. SWIMMING **445**
12. STRENGTH TRAINING **508**
13. JUMPING ROPE **508**
14. PLAYING ULTIMATE FRISBEE **508**
15. ROAD RUNNING **508**
16. MOUNTAIN BIKING ON HILLY TERRAIN **540**
17. TRAIL RUNNING HILLS **572**
18. RUNNING IN SAND **597**
19. PLAYING SOCCER .... **445 - 635**
20. CYCLING VIGOROUSLY UPHILL .... **508 - 635**
21. BOULDERING **699**
22. ROWING .... **445 - 762**
23. RUNNING UP STAIRS **953**

Source: *Compendium of Physical Activities Tracking Guide*

body wants to use incoming carbohydrates to restore the glycogen that was depleted during your workout. So the carbs you eat after exercise get stored in your muscles, not in your spare tire.

But it gets better: Your body—which is still burning calories at an advanced rate hours after you finish your workout—is now desperate to come up with energy to keep your brain thinking and your heart beating and your fingernails growing. And since all the food you're eating is being stored in your muscles, your body has to start hunting around for something else to burn. Oh, here's something I can burn: belly fat!

And because aerobic exercise calls on glycogen, too, incorporating a bit of aerobic exercise into your weight routine can enhance that effect. A study in the *British Journal of Nutrition* found that after 90 minutes of moderate-intensity cycling, a postexercise meal of nearly a pound of pasta (400 grams of cooked pasta, yielding 297 grams of carbs) resulted in zero fat creation. You read that right—a pound of pasta and no fat creation. All of those carbs were shuttled back into the muscles for later use. That's why the *Women's Health* Fast-Track Tone-Up Plan keeps you working quickly and efficiently, triggering an aerobic burn and a muscle burn.

A major bonus of the *Women's Health* Fast-Track Tone-Up Plan: You get to eat some of your favorite food before and after your workout. In fact, your post-workout meal might be your most indulgent meal of the day. You can eat more calories and even enjoy a little something sweet: Research shows that a combination of carbohydrates (some from sugar) and protein is the best concoction for speeding muscle growth. A superfast, supercheap answer: chocolate milk. Sure, there are plenty of expensive recovery shakes

> **HOT TIP #74**
>
> **Double your abs.** Canadian researchers determined that your abs work nearly twice as hard when you do a plank with your feet on a Swiss ball instead of on the floor.

for sale at your gym, but more than five research universities have concluded that the stuff you drank in fourth grade remains the ultimate muscle-nourishing cocktail. So grab a straw and slurp it down!

Why Upping Your Metabolism Is Easier Than You Think

Even before you start exercising, there are still plenty of tricks you can use to eliminate visceral fat, improve your flab-burning metabolic process, and start losing weight fast.

1. DON'T DIET

The *Women's Health* Diet isn't about eating less; it's about eating more—more nutrient-dense food, to crowd out the empty calories and keep you full all day. That's important, because restricting food will kill your metabolism. It sends a signal to your body that says, "I'm starving here!" And your body responds by slowing your metabolic rate to hold on to existing energy stores. What's worse, if the food shortage (meaning, your crash diet) continues, you'll begin burning muscle tissue, which just gives your enemy, visceral fat, a greater advantage. Your metabolism slows further, and fat goes on to claim even more territory.

2. GO TO BED EARLIER

A study in Finland looked at sets of identical twins and discovered that in each set of siblings, the twin who slept less and was under more stress had more visceral fat.

3. EAT MORE PROTEIN

Your body needs protein to maintain lean muscle. In a 2006 article in the *American Journal of Clinical Nutrition,* researchers argued that the current recommended daily intake for protein, 0.36 grams per pound of body weight, is woefully inadequate for anyone doing resistance training and recommend that women get between 0.54 and 1 gram per pound of body weight. (If you want to lose weight, use your goal body weight as your guide.) Add a serving, like 3 ounces of lean meat, 2 tablespoons of nuts, or 8 ounces of low-fat yogurt, to every meal and snack. Plus, research shows that protein can up postmeal calorie burn by as much as 35 percent.

4. GO ORGANIC WHEN YOU CAN

Canadian researchers report that dieters with the most organo-chlorines (pollutants from pesticides, which are stored in fat cells) experience a greater-than-normal dip in metabolism as they lose weight, perhaps because the toxins interfere with the energy-burning process. In other words, pesticides make it harder to lose pounds. Of course, it's not always easy to find—or afford—organic produce. But in general, conventionally grown items that you peel—avocado, grapefruit, bananas—are fine. But choose organic when buying celery, peaches, strawberries, apples, blueberries, nectarines, sweet bell peppers, spinach, kale and collard greens, cherries, potatoes, and imported grapes; they tend to have the highest levels of pesticides.

> **HOT TIP #75**
>
> **Sprout a healthy new diet.** Baby broccoli sprouts have 100 times as much cancer-fighting sulforaphane as mature broccoli.

5. GET UP, STAND UP

Whether you sit or stand at work may play as big a role in your waistline as your fitness routine. Missouri University researchers discovered that inactivity (4 hours or more) causes a near shutdown of an enzyme that controls fat and cholesterol metabolism.

To keep this enzyme active and increase your fat-burning, break up long periods of downtime by standing up—for example, while talking on the phone.

6. DRINK COLD WATER

German researchers found that drinking 6 cups of cold water a day (that's 48 ounces) can raise resting metabolism by about 50 calories daily—enough to shed 5 pounds in a year, with essentially zero additional effort. The increase may come from the work it takes to heat the water to body temperature.

7. EAT THE HEAT

It turns out that capsaicin, the compound that gives chile peppers their heat, can also fire up your metabolism. Eating about 1 tablespoon of chopped peppers (red or green) boosts your sympathetic nervous system (responsible for your fight-or-flight response), according to a

Measure your metabolic rate

The best way to measure your daily metabolic rate is to log all the foods and liquids you ingest daily for a minimum of 3 days. (Try the USDA's online tool http://www.mypyramidtracker.gov). If you're not gaining weight, then your daily calorie consumption is also your metabolic rate. If you're packing on the pounds, your metabolic rate is lower than your calorie intake and you need to tweak your eating habits.

If food logs aren't for you, gyms and health clubs usually have devices that assess your metabolic rate. The Bod Pod, for example, has sensors that measure the air your body displaces when you sit in it. The machine uses that information to determine your muscle-to-fat ratio. (To find one near you, go to bodpod.com).

study published in the *Journal of Nutritional Science and Vitaminology*. The result: a temporary metabolism spike of about 23 percent. Stock up on chile peppers to add to salsas, and keep a jar of red-pepper flakes on hand for topping pizzas, pastas, and stir-fries.

8. REV UP IN THE MORNING

Eating breakfast jump-starts your metabolism so it's no accident that those who skip this meal are 4½ times as likely to be obese. The heartier your first meal is, the better. In one study published by the *American Journal of Epidemiology*, volunteers who got 22 to 55 percent of their total calories at breakfast gained only 1.7 pounds on average over 4 years. While those who got zero to 11 percent gained nearly 3 pounds.

> **HOT TIP #76**
>
> **Coffee it up.**
> Athletes who drink caffeine before exercise have 66 percent more glycogen in their muscles, giving them greater endurance.

9. DRINK COFFEE OR TEA

Caffeine is a central nervous system stimulant, so your daily java jolts can rev your metabolism by 5 to 8 percent—burning about 98 to 174 calories a day. A cup of brewed tea can raise your metabolism by 12 percent, according to one Japanese study. Researchers believe antioxidants called catechins in tea provide the boost.

10. FIGHT FAT WITH FIBER

Research shows that some fiber can fire up your fat burn by as much as 30 percent. Studies find that those who eat the most fiber gain the least weight over time. Aim for about 25 grams a day—the amount in about three servings each of fruits and vegetables.

11. EAT IRON-RICH FOODS

Iron is essential for carrying the oxygen your muscles need to burn fat. Unless you restock your stores, you run the risk of low energy and a sagging metabolism. Shellfish, lean meats, beans, fortified cereals, and spinach are excellent sources.

12. GET MORE VITAMIN D

Vitamin D is essential for preserving muscle tissue. Get 90 percent of your recommended daily intake (400 IU) in a 3.5-ounce serving of salmon. Other good sources: tuna, fortified milk and cereal, and eggs.

13. DRINK MILK

There's some evidence that calcium deficiency, which is common in many women, may slow metabolism. Research shows that consuming calcium through dairy foods such as fat-free milk and low-fat yogurt may also reduce fat absorption from other foods.

14. EAT WATERMELON

The amino acid arginine, abundant in watermelon, might promote weight loss, according to the *Journal of Nutrition*. In a laboratory study, adding this amino acid to the diet of obese mice enhanced the oxidation of fat and glucose. Snack on watermelon and other arginine sources, such as seafood, nuts, and seeds, year-round.

HOT TIP #77

Eat melons, skip melanoma. One slice of watermelon contains up to 10 milligrams of cancer-fighting lycopene—as much as four tomatoes.

15. STAY HYDRATED

All of your body's chemical reactions, including your metabolism, depend on water. If you are dehydrated, you may be burning up to 2 percent fewer calories, according to researchers at the University of Utah. Drink at least eight to twelve 8-ounce glasses a day.

A pound of
body fat only burns
2 calories a day,
while a pound
of skeletal muscles
burns 6 calories
a day.

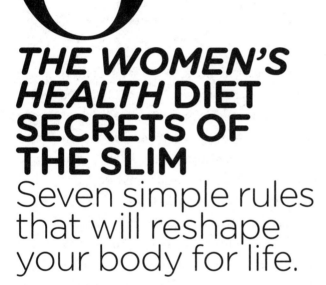

THE WOMEN'S HEALTH DIET SECRETS OF THE SLIM
Seven simple rules that will reshape your body for life.

We at *Women's Health* have had our fair share of struggles with the scale. But we've also benefited from our unique access to the most scientific, up-to-date body of knowledge about weight loss on the planet. It's this kind of authoritative research that has gone into creating the founding principles of the *Women's Health Diet*, which we can't wait to share with you. We call them the Secrets of the Slim. Think of them as seven insider tips that make it easier to lose weight. Not that you're going to have to abide by them every day—you're not, and neither do our editors. But the closer you adhere to them, the faster you'll reach your ideal physique. Consider them pledges—pledges to yourself. You're going to be amazed at just how easy they are to stick to.

Why the Secrets of the Slim will work for you

As we said at the beginning of this book, there's a war going on inside your body, a war between fat and muscle. But in this eternal battle, fat has the advantage. And for that, you can blame Mother Nature.

When humans first evolved, starvation and deprivation were always a threat. So our bodies learned to store fat in lean times and to burn fewer calories when calories weren't easy to come by—just as bears do when preparing for hibernation.

The problem is that today we no longer have to scratch our way across the savanna, looking for grubs to eat. Today we are surrounded by grub to eat, stacked on 18-foot-high shelves at the local grocery store. And yet, strangely, we still put our bodies in starvation mode more than we might expect. We skip breakfast to race to our jobs. We work long days, breaking to eat only when our bellies rumble. Sometimes, we even go on diets, trying to earn some sort of merit badge by depriving ourselves.

But every time you skip a meal or feel a hunger pang? Your body feels it, too, and says, "Uh-oh. Famine up ahead. Better shuttle some of those potato chips down into the belly for good measure."

Literally, every time you let yourself grow hungry, you're telling your body to store fat. That's why each of our Secrets of the Slim is designed to keep you eating—a lot. To melt away fat and build new muscle, you'll need to eat nutrient-rich foods that are both filling and delicious throughout the day. As you'll discover, all of the guidelines of the *Women's Health* Nutrition System are about eating more food, not depriving yourself of it. Your goal is to pack your body with so much good nutrition that it forgets about the junk calories out there and instead starts to build and maintain new muscle and shed flab. To help you achieve your ideal body, you'll focus on goal-driven eating that eliminates the need to count calories. In fact, we've made this plan insanely flexible by giving you an easy-to-digest breakdown of eight key food groups—you'll meet them in the next chapter—and a wide variety of ways to enjoy and indulge in them.

HOT TIP #78

Tune into yellowfin.
Yellowfin tuna carries mercury levels that are up to 50 percent lower than those of bluefin or bigeye.

But first, you need to know the Secrets of the Slim. As you commit them to memory, you'll discover that when you eat is almost as important as what you eat. As you begin to work with your body's natural metabolic clock, you'll be shocked at how easy it is to lose and how fast our plan begins to take effect.

SLIM SECRET #1:
"I Will Eat Protein With Every Meal and Every Snack."

Here's why this rule is so important: At any given moment, even at rest, your body is breaking down and building up protein, says Jeffrey Volek, PhD, RD, of the University of Connecticut. Substitute the word "protein" for "muscle" and you quickly understand just how dynamic your body is and how your muscle content can change considerably in the course of just a few weeks.

But muscle doesn't come simply from lifting weights or hauling groceries up the stairs. Eating protein triggers muscle growth. In fact, every time you eat at least 10 to 15 grams of protein, you trigger a burst of protein synthesis. And when you eat at least 30 grams, that period of synthesis lasts about 3 hours—and that means even more muscle growth. Here's a quick look at what those numbers translate into when they actually hit your plate:

30 Grams of Protein	10 to 15 Grams of Protein
1 4-oz hamburger patty	1 fruit-and-yogurt parfait w/ granola
1 large chicken breast	2 medium carrots w/ ½ cup hummus
1 4-oz sirloin steak	¾ cup chili con carne
1 3-egg vegetable omelet with 3 strips bacon	10-oz spaghetti w/meat sauce
20 large peel-and-eat wild shrimp	1 pouch chunk light tuna
1 lobster	½ cup oatmeal w/ 1 cup 2% milk
1 haddock filet	12 oz lowfat chocolate milk
1 6-oz pork chop	6 oz Greek yogurt
1 6-oz serving tempeh	2 Tbsp peanut butter on whole wheat

Now think about it: When would you typically eat most of your protein? At dinner, right? That means you might be fueling your muscles for only a few hours a day, mostly while you're watching *Chelsea Lately*. The rest of the day, you're breaking down muscle, because you don't have enough protein in your system. "The single most important diet upgrade for people who want to lose weight is to eat protein for breakfast," says Louis Aronne, MD, director of the Comprehensive Weight Control Program at New York–Presbyterian Hospital/ Weill Cornell Medical Center. "I've had clients lose a bunch of weight just by making this one change." (It's weight-loss magic, especially when you focus on eating protein at breakfast: In one study, overweight subjects ate the same number of calories for breakfast, but one group got their calories from eggs, the second group from bagels.

After 8 weeks, the egg eaters lost 65 percent more weight—and showed no increase in cholesterol or triglycerides.)

YOUR PLAN: Eat protein at all three meals, which can include meats and eggs or other options such as cheese and milk. You need to boost your protein intake to between .54 and 1 gram per pound of body weight to preserve your calorie-burning muscle mass. (That's a total of between 76 and 140 grams daily for a 140-pound woman.)

Important note: We said *goal* bodyweight. Why is that a big deal? Well, if you calculate your protein intake based on your current weight, you may not see the scale budge. Say you weigh 150 pounds and want to lose 20 pounds. Your goal bodyweight would be 130 pounds and you'd want to aim for anywhere between 70 and 130 grams of protein per day. That translates to roughly 30 grams of protein at your main meals, with filling options like a chicken breast, a hamburger patty,

> **HOT TIP #79**
>
> **Count on Chocula.** As few as 30 calories a day of dark chocolate can help lower blood pressure.

or a filet of fish. For snacks, eat at least 10 to 15 grams of protein, such as two hard-boiled eggs, an order of rice and beans, or even a classic peanut butter and jelly sandwich on wheat bread. And when in doubt, reach for milk or cheese. Harvard Medical School researchers found that people who ate three servings of dairy food daily (1,200 milligrams of calcium) were 60 percent less likely to be overweight than people who consumed fewer servings.

TRICK YOURSELF SLIM: Make a snack out of yogurt once a day. Not only does it provide a calcium hit, but a University of Tennessee study found that people who added three servings of yogurt a day to their diet lost 81 percent more belly fat over 12 weeks than those who didn't eat yogurt. And a study in the journal *Molecular Systems Biology* found that yogurt-based bacteria can prevent the body from absorbing fat.

SLIM SECRET #2:

"I Will Never Eat the World's Worst Breakfast."

What's the world's worst breakfast?

No breakfast at all.

When you wake up in the morning, your body is fuel-deprived. It's been 7 to 9 hours (or more) since you last ate. Your insulin levels have dropped, your protein stores are empty, and your muscles are desperate for nutrition. Your body needs food to restore its balance. "The bulk of your calories should come at breakfast," says David Grotto, RD, national spokesperson for the American Dietetic Association. "When you shift calories to the morning, you lose weight and keep it off." If you skip breakfast, you lower your metabolism, starve your muscles, and wind up eating the bulk of your calories too late in the day. That's why regularly skipping breakfast increases your risk of obesity by 450 percent.

Breakfast is the one meal where, calories be damned, eating more is almost always better than eating less—in an ideal world, you'd get between 500 and 600 calories at breakfast alone. Just make sure some of those calories come from protein: In a 2008 study, researchers at Virginia Commonwealth University found that people who regularly ate a protein-rich 600-calorie breakfast lost significantly more weight in 8 months than those who consumed only 300 calories and a quarter of the protein. The big-breakfast eaters lost an average of 40 pounds and had an easier time sticking with the diet even though both groups were prescribed about the same number of total daily calories.

And that's why the world's worst breakfast is no breakfast at all.

> **HOT TIP #80**
>
> **Reach the beach.**
> A stroll on the sand uses more than 2½ times as much energy as regular walking, and builds greater calf strength.

Okay, class, we can tell some of you are getting anxious. Or maybe you're thinking, *I know something worse than nothing for breakfast*. Well, we doubt it. Breakfast is like a paycheck: Lousy is always better than nothing. Go ahead, just try to come up with a breakfast that's worth skipping...

HOW ABOUT ... a sugar donut?! Definitely not the ideal breakfast solution, but ... a Sugar-Raised Donut at Dunkin' Donuts is only 190 calories, and with it you're still getting a little protein (3 grams). Add a glass of milk and now you've raised your protein and lowered your percentage of sugar, and you're still under 350 calories. (Caveat: We don't recommend making a habit of the doughnut breakfast.)

HOW ABOUT ... a cup of joe and an Egg McMuffin? *Sooo* much better than nothing at all. In fact, the much-maligned McMuffin actually deserves props as one of the few fast-food options with more protein (18 grams) than fat (12 grams).

GOTCHA NOW ... a couple of slices of leftover pizza! You're getting pretty desperate here, but okay. Two slices of Domino's Hand-Tossed Cheese and Pepperoni rack up about 510 calories and 22 grams of fat. But you've got 22 grams of protein from the meat and cheese, calcium from the cheese, carbs for energy from the crust, and even a few vitamins from the tomato sauce. Now consider that in a 2010 study in the *International Journal of Obesity*, the subjects who consumed the most protein at breakfast ate 130 fewer calories at a subsequent lunch than those who consumed the least protein.

HOT TIP #81

Make it sweeter without sweets. People on low-sugar diets have less depression and anxiety than carb consumers.

WHAT IF ... you took a whole cinnamon bun, fried it, then slathered it in cream cheese, stuffed it with maple-syrup ice cream, and doused it in caramel? Okay, you're really stretching here. What twisted mind could create such a monstrosity? Oh, Friendly's did? And it's on their breakfast menu? And it's called Caramel Cinnamon Swirl French Toast? Okay, you've got us with this one. At 2,090 calories, it's more than most of us need to eat per day. Plus, a mind-blowing 856 of them come from sugar! Then you've got 57 grams of fat, half a day's sodium intake, and minimal protein. Wow, that really is the world's worst breakfast.

Conclusion: If you are shipwrecked on a deserted island and the only thing left standing from the now-extinct former civilization is an abandoned Friendly's, and the dust-enshrouded freezer unit has just one thing left to eat and it's Caramel Cinnamon Swirl French Toast . . . well, in that case, you're excused from breakfast.

Otherwise, wake up and start eating!

HOT TIP #82

Hangover cure #397. Amino acids in poached eggs help erase next-day hurtin', according to a study in the *Journal of Inflammation Research.*

YOUR PLAN: Eat a large portion of your daily calories—30 to 35 percent of your total intake—in the morning. The very best breakfast will match proteins and whole grains with produce and healthy fats. For example: eggs over easy on whole-grain toast and a protein-and-fruit smoothie. If you have neither the time nor the stomach for a big breakfast, eat two small ones—have cereal with your coffee, then grab a yogurt and fruit to eat at your desk. But the bottom line is this: Get some protein for breakfast, and the rest of the day will take care of itself.

TRICK YOURSELF SLIM: Absolutely, positively, zero time to have anything but a cup of coffee? Okay: Before you pour the coffee, fill your cup with milk. Drink it down until you have just the right amount to lighten your joe, then add the caffeine. Eight ounces of 1 percent milk gives you 110 calories and 8 grams of protein, along with a hit of fat-burning calcium. Even if you can't possibly eat breakfast, well, guess what: You just ate breakfast!

SLIM SECRET #3:
"I Will Eat Before and After Exercise."

As with romance, comedy, and the stock market, timing is everything when it comes to food and exercise. And the great news if you love to eat: You probably need to eat more. In fact, eating more of the right foods at the right time can turn every workout into the best workout of your life.

Nowadays researchers are worrying a lot less about what you eat and how you sweat, and thinking a lot more about when you do both. Here's what eating at the right time can do for you:

BUILD LEAN MUSCLE! Eating before a workout speeds muscle growth, according to Dutch and British researchers. In one study, subjects who ate a protein- and carbohydrate-rich snack right before and right after their workouts fueled their muscles twice as effectively as those who waited at least 5 hours to eat. By feeding your body with protein and carbohydrates within an hour or two of exercise, you provide your muscles with enough energy to build strength and burn fat more effectively.

BURN MORE FAT. Syracuse University researchers found that when you down protein before and after weight training, you blunt the effects of cortisol, the stress hormone that tells your body to store fat. As a result, you burn more fat not only during your workout but also for an additional 24 hours afterward. (Study participants ate a combo of 22 grams of protein and 35 grams of carbs—about what you'd get from a glass of milk and a peanut butter and jelly sandwich.)

SCULPT YOUR BODY AND MAKE YOU LOOK YOUNGER! Finnish scientists who had weight lifters drink a protein shake before and after a workout discovered that

HOT TIP #83

Cow the dentist. Eating yogurt four times a week reduces your risk of cavities by 25 percent.

their subjects produced more of a molecule called cyclin-dependent kinase 2 (CDK2). This molecule signals your muscles to produce more stem cells, which aid the process of building muscle and improve your body's ability to heal after resistance training. Stem cells are your body's microscopic fountains of youth: The shake drinkers not only gained more muscle than their counterparts; they also had a higher muscle-to-flab ratio than those who didn't drink the shakes.

HOT TIP #84

Get clean, get lean. You don't need liposuction to vacuum off the fat. In an Indiana University study, people with the cleanest houses had the highest levels of physical activity. "It could be that these people burn a lot of extra calories keeping their homes clean," says study author NiCole Keith, PhD.

FEEL MORE ENERGY—AND LESS PAIN! British researchers discovered that eating a mix of protein and carbs before and after your workout can inhibit muscle breakdown and reduce inflammation. That means you both replace fat with muscle faster and you recover more quickly, with less next-day soreness.

All this just from eating a little more food? Now, that's a diet!

YOUR PLAN: Eat a snack containing carbohydrates and protein 30 minutes or so before your workout and one of your protein-rich meals immediately after. (At *Women's Health* we often say, "Lost time is lost muscle." Your body breaks down muscle during and after exercise to use as fuel, and it rebuilds muscle using calories that you've consumed. The longer you wait after exercise to eat, the more your body will break down its own muscle and the less it will build new muscle.

TRICK YOURSELF SLIM: A protein shake right after your shower is one of the fastest nutrition delivery systems there is. You can even download our *Women's Health* Smoothie Selector app at www.menshealth.com/apps.

SLIM SECRET #4:
"I Will Eat It If It Grows on a Tree."

Or a bush, stalk, or vine, as well. In other words, if it grows on or is a plant, eat it. Fruits and vegetables should be included in every meal and in as many snacks as you can. The reason: Your goal is to fill your body with as many muscle-promoting, fat-discouraging nutrients as possible, and the very best sources of them are fruits, nuts, and vegetables. By providing your body with the maximum amount of nutrients for the least number of calories, they're a dietary bargain. A study at UCLA found that the typical person of normal weight consumed two servings of fruit a day, on average, while the typical overweight person ate just one serving. Another study in the journal *Appetite* found that eating whole fruit at the beginning of a meal reduces your overall calorie intake by 15 percent. Now, a caveat: Eating "vegetable chips" or "veggie sticks" or drinking "fruit-flavored punch" is not the same thing. If the fruit or vegetable in question won't wilt after a few days of hanging out on your countertop or in your fridge, then it's a processed food. It didn't grow on a tree; it grew out of some scientist's imagination.

Another benefit to eating off the trees: You'll get more heart-healthy omega-3 fatty acids. Some experts argue that omega-3s should be labeled essential nutrients, as necessary to health as, say, vitamins A and D. "They're involved in the metabolism of each individual cell," says Artemis P. Simopoulos, MD, the president of the Center for Genetics, Nutrition and Health, in Washington, D.C. "They're part of your body's basic nutrition." Studies show that this healthy fat may not only reduce a person's risk of heart disease and stroke but may also help prevent ailments as diverse as Alzheimer's disease, arthritis, asthma, attention deficit disorder, and autoimmune disorders—and those are just the A's. Plus, on top of their mood-boosting, heart-saving, brain-enhancing powers, omega-3-rich foods help those who consume a lot of them live longer and carry less abdominal fat. And scientists from Quebec found that omega-3s improve protein metabolism, meaning that more of the protein you eat is synthesized in your muscle. Sure, it sounds cool, but even better, this means your muscles will respond faster. You already know that you can find this healthy fat in fish such as salmon and tuna, but it's also found growing in trees: Two highly potent sources of omega-3s are walnuts and kiwifruit. (Keep a container of ground flaxseed in your kitchen as well; this seed is extremely high in omega-3s and adds a nutty flavor to smoothies, PB&J sandwiches, and salads.)

HOT TIP #85

Envision success. University of Iowa scientists found that people who monitored their diet and exercise goals most frequently were more likely to achieve them than people who set goals but rarely reviewed them.

YOUR PLAN: Eat at least one serving of fruits or vegetables at every meal. You can and should eat as any fruits and vegetables as you want to help satisfy cravings.

TRICK YOURSELF SLIM: Eat your fruits and vegetables first! Not only will you consume more vegetables and fewer calories from other foods, but the fiber content will lower the glycemic load of your meal as well, helping you sidestep those swings in blood sugar that lead to hunger. Try at least one new fruit or vegetable each week, and make sure that salads and fruit salads have at least four different colors. For example: lettuce, yellow peppers, tomatoes, and carrots; or pineapple, blood oranges, kiwi, and grapes.

SLIM SECRET #5:
"I Will Become a Salad Savant."

Women are lucky. We don't have to skulk around hiding our salad habit from our friends the way guys think they do. We are free to embrace greens in all their nutritional glory. Problem is, we don't. According to a recent *Eating Patterns in America* report, issued by the market research group NPD, just 17 percent of home-prepared dinners include salad, down from 22 percent in 1994. And when we eat out, it's even worse: Salads make up just 5 percent of the main courses we order.

The "house salad" has become our default. (As in, "I'll have the house salad. Oil and vinegar on the side.")

Well, ladies. It's time to paddle yourself off that iceberg-studded channel and get your feet wet with—wait for it—better-for-you bowls of goodness.

The reason is that salads deliver wildly important nutrients that are hard to come by elsewhere—nutrients that help promote weight loss. And you get more of these nutrients when you partake of a wide variety of ingredients.

Example number one: Folate, a B vitamin found primarily in leafy greens, is perhaps the best indicator of how healthy your diet really is. Folate deficiency is linked to most of the major diseases of our time. It leads to an increased risk of stroke, heart disease, obesity, cognitive impairment, Alzheimer's disease, cancer, and depression, as well as to a decreased response to depression treatments. Some of the best food sources of folate are foods you're not going to eat a lot of, no matter how much you're told—kale, Swiss chard, and collard greens. Had any lately?

> **HOT TIP #86**
>
> **Sip up, sit up.**
> You can do 17 percent more reps when you're well-hydrated, say researchers at the University of Connecticut.

127

No? Then it's all the more important that when you order a salad, you lean whenever possible toward mixed greens, spinach, or endive. It's hard to get enough folate (other sources are broccoli, brussels sprouts, lentils, beans, liver, and peas— again, not exactly a roll call of all-time favorite foods), but it's worth it: A study in the *British Journal of Nutrition* found that dieters who ate the most folate were able to lose 8.5 times as much weight as those who ate the least.

> **HOT TIP #87**
>
> **Chew through the fat.** In one study, women who were asked to eat quickly consumed more food (in less time) than those who were told to eat slowly. The women who were told to slow down chewed each bite 15 to 20 times and paused before taking the next bite.

YOUR PLAN: At every meal, try to include a folate-rich food. The best way to up your folate intake is to eat leafy greens with as many meals as you can, and eat them first.

TRICK YOURSELF SLIM: Boost your salad's power with a dressing made from mustard, vinegar, and safflower oil. In a study in the *American Journal of Clinical Nutrition*, researchers found that the high amounts of linoleic acid in safflower oil may keep your body from storing fat.

SLIM SECRET #6:
"I Will Not Drink Sugar Water."

This sounds like the most obvious secret of all, right? After all, when was the last time you drank sugar water?

If you're like most Americans, the answer is . . . earlier today. A recent study in the *American Journal of Clinical Nutrition* showed that around 37 percent of our total daily liquid calories come from sugar-sweetened drinks. Which are, drumroll please, nothing more than sugar and water with flavor and color thrown in. Here are some common sugar waters that you might have enjoyed recently:

COLA: SUGAR WATER + CARAMEL COLORING AND FLAVORING
A typical cola is about 89 percent carbonated water and 9 percent high-fructose corn syrup.

SWEETENED ICED TEA: SUGAR WATER + TEA
Teas like Snapple are about 89 percent water and 10 percent high–fructose corn syrup.

VITAMIN WATER: SUGAR WATER + CHEMICAL FORMS OF VITAMINS
One of the worst things to happen to both water and vitamins: An average brand is 92 percent water and more than 5 percent sugar.

FRUIT DRINKS: SUGAR WATER + FRUIT JUICE
If your juice has the word "cocktail" attached to it, it's about 63 percent water, 27 percent juice, and more than 9 percent high-fructose corn syrup.

ENERGY DRINKS: SUGAR WATER + CAFFEINE AND HERBS
Though they list plenty of mysterious ingredients, like taurine and guarana and milk thistle, the average energy drink is 84.5 percent water and 12.3 percent sugar.

In fact, the average American now drinks more than 450 calories every day. By cutting that amount in half—which you could do simply by eliminating sugar water from your diet—you would cut enough calories to lose about 25 pounds in a year. Plus, you'd eliminate one of biggest sources of fructose, a component in most types of sweeteners that's coming under more scrutiny every year. In 2010, Robert Lustig, MD, professor of clinical pediatrics at the University of California, San Francisco, discovered that fructose has much the same effect on the human body as alcohol does, including causing the same kind of liver scarring as is found in alcoholics.

YOUR PLAN: Replace sodas, iced teas, and "performance beverages" with water, seltzer, or other low-calorie or calorie-free beverages. (And don't just change over to the "diet" version of your favorite soft drink. You'll read why in a few minutes.) If you don't like the taste of your water, buy a home filter tap, which will help take out any chemical tastes, and keep a container of it cold in your fridge. Researchers from the University of Utah found that people who drink the most water have the fastest metabolisms. In a study, subjects drank 4, 8, or 12 cups of water each day. Those who drank at least 8 cups reported better concentration and higher energy levels, and tests showed that they were burning calories at a much higher rate than the 4-cup-a-day group.

TRICK YOURSELF SLIM: A study in the *Journal of the American Dietetic Association* found that drinking a glass of water before breakfast can cut daily food intake by 13 percent. So on top of the calories you're saving by swapping soda for H_2O, you're saving another 200 or so by staving off hunger pangs! (That's another 21 pounds gone in a year!)

A CAVEAT: You'd think the easiest way to cut out sugar-water calories would be to switch to diet sodas and teas. And yes, that will cut calories. But for reasons we don't fully grasp, diet sodas actually increase your risk of weight gain. Research shows that people who drink one to two cans of regular soda per day increase their risk of becoming overweight or obese by nearly 33 percent. But replace those regular sodas with diet sodas and the risk rises to 65 percent more likely to become overweight and 41 percent more likely to become obese. Several studies have hinted at why this is. In 2009, Purdue University researchers found that artificial sweeteners may interfere with your brain's satisfaction signals, essentially making you crave more food than you need. And even more recent research by scientists in the Department of Psychological Sciences at Purdue suggests that artificial sweeteners may slow metabolism—meaning the more diet soda you drink, the fewer calories you burn during the day. And because artificial sweeteners are 200 to 2,000 times sweeter than sugar, stirring a teaspoonful into your daily cup of joe may mean that when you do use real sugar, it just doesn't taste sweet enough for you, making you grab for extra sugar packets.

> **HOT TIP #88**
>
> **Make a pit stop.** Natural anti-inflammatories in olives suppress the same pain pathways as over-the counter ibuprofen.

SLIM SECRET #7:

"I Will Follow the Secrets of the Slim ~~100 Percent~~ 80 Percent of the Time."

If you make the right food choices 80 percent of the time, you can't help but get—and stay—lean. That means that one out of every five times you make a choice about what to put in your mouth, you get a free pass to make a lame one. Like that baby shower where the host hands you a piece of cake and insists you eat it. Or that girls' night out involving one too many parasol-festooned cocktails. It happens, because nobody's perfect—and not trying to be perfect is one of the keys to long-term success. Those of us who try to be perfect eventually go crazy, and the next thing you know, they're wearing a GPS monitoring device on their ankles and writing not-so-friendly messages to judges on their fingernails. Don't let that happen to you.

YOUR PLAN: Don't try to be perfect. Be 80 percent. That'll still put you well ahead of the rest of the population. But when you do cheat, cheat with the best. In Chapter 10, you'll find a list of the 250 best foods for women. If you want a chocolate bar, go ahead—but make sure it's the best one. (That would be Dagoba's Organic Beacoup Berries bar, which mixes in cherries and cranberries to pack a whopping 7 grams of fiber for just 250 calories.) Craving a steak? Go get one, but make the very best choice. (At Ruby Tuesday, you can order a plain-grilled top sirloin with just 391 calories—ordering it "plain" will strip off 1,000 milligrams of sodium.) Make a peanut butter and jelly sandwich, but use only the best PB and the best J (see page 223), and the best bread in the world. (All the best choices for every craving are in Chapter 10.)

You'll be stunned at how effective this strategy is. Let's look at a potential three-day menu: Say, for instance, that Friday night you gave in and ordered a burger at a chain restaurant; on

Saturday night, your guy convinced you to go out for ribs (yeah, they're messy, but they melt in your mouth, right?); and on Sunday night, you heated up a frozen pizza while catching up on Facebook. Each of the three mornings you had a bowl of cereal, and lunch was a modest cup of yogurt and a piece of fruit. Here's what the difference might be if you ate the very best food, instead of the worst:

BEST	WORST	SAVINGS
BURGER McDonald's Big N' Tasty (hold the mayo) 410 calories	Cheesecake Factory Ranch House Burger 1,941 calories	**1,531 calories**
RIBS (½ RACK) Ruby Tuesday's Memphis- Dry Rub Fork-Tender 460 calories	Applebee's Double-Glazed Baby Back Ribs 1,000 calories	**540 calories**
FROZEN PIZZA (⅓ PIE) Amy's Cheese Pizza 290 calories	DiGiorno for One, Traditional Crust Supreme Pizza 790 calories	**500 calories**
CEREAL Kashi Whole-Wheat Biscuits, Cinnamon Harvest 180 calories	Quaker Natural Granola with Raisins 420 calories	**240 calories (x3!)**
YOGURT Stonyfield Farm Oikos Organic Greek Yogurt, Plain 80 calories	Yoplait Strawberry Original 99% Fat Free 170 calories	**90 calories (x3!)**
Total calories saved in just one weekend		**3,561!**

Now consider this: It takes 3,500 calories to build a pound of fat. In just 72 hours, by eating the exact same food, just better versions of the same, you could actually save more than a pound of fat! Do that every weekend for a year—and remember, you're still eating yummy stuff like burgers and pizza—and you could shed 52 pounds of flab. (And that's without even changing how you eat on weekdays!)

Amazing, right? Make the right choice 80 percent of the time, and you'll have this fat thing solved. More than 80 percent? You'll be downright Aniston-esque.

TRICK YOURSELF SLIM: If you eat something that's really, truly horrible for you (like, you can't stop thinking about the Friendly's Caramel Cinnamon Swirl French Toast, wash it down with a glass of milk. A study in the *American Journal of Clinical Nutrition* found that those who consume calcium from dairy every day decrease the triacylglycerol levels in the blood (a major form fat in the blood) by 15 to 19 percent.

A Word About Counting Calories

No matter how healthy you eat, consuming more calories than your body burns is a surefire route to weight gain. That's why many diet plans are based on counting calories, using very tightly managed caloric calculations to ensure that dieters never go over their allotted food intake.

At *Women's Health*, we've spent nearly a decade studying calorie-counting systems—using the absolute best science and soliciting the finest mathematical minds—and boiling these intensely intricate scientific findings into an equation anyone can understand. The ultimate calorie-intake formula for women looks like this:

**Caloric intake
x
BMI²
÷
waist circumference
−
(3,500 ÷ (24 + 7))
=
$%#*&@ BORING!**

Look, we know you're busy. Who wants to whip out a calculator each time you sit down to a well-deserved meal? It's far more effective in the long run to train your brain to recognize correct portion sizes so you learn to eat mindfully.

It's going to take a little practice, because over the past 30 years, food marketers have tricked out their offerings, burying normal-size servings in biggie sizes and "extra-value" meals that don't look at all like portions are supposed to. The problem is most egregious at America's restaurants, where they now market meal-size plates as appetizers, family-size platters as single entrées, and small kiddie pools as beverages. A 2008 study by the USDA found that Americans consume an average of 107 more calories each time they go to a restaurant. And a 2002 study looking at restaurant portions found that the average restaurant pasta dish was nearly five times bigger than the USDA's recommended serving! Steaks and bagels were more than three times as big, and hamburgers more than double.

So how can the average woman defend herself against calorie counts and serving sizes that are ballooning faster than the national debt? How can you become a nutritional Tea Party of one, cutting down on excess caloric spending while still getting the fat, protein, fiber, and other nutrients you need? And how can you do it all the same way you pick out a new nail polish—by eyeballing it? The answer is in the palm of your hand. Literally. For solid foods, a serving size is equal to:

MEATS: The size of your palm

VEGETABLES AND FRUITS: The size of a tight fist

OILS AND OTHER HEALTHY FATS: A teaspoon is equal to the end of your thumb from the knuckle up

NUTS, BEANS, AND LEGUMES: Whatever fits in the palm of your hand

GRAINS: The size of a tight fist

DAIRY: The size of your palm

By reading labels and staying clear of beverages with added sugars, you will cut calories, shed pounds, and reprogram your taste buds so they will stop craving sweet foods and drinks. Then you can devote your sweet tooth to treats that should be sweet, like chocolate, berries, and ice cream.

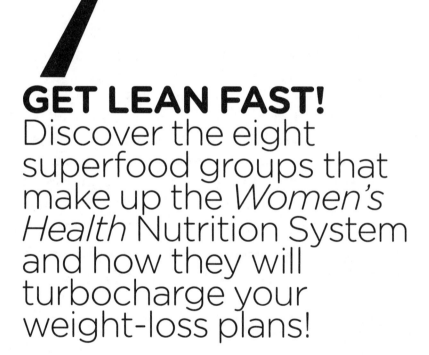

GET LEAN FAST!

Discover the eight superfood groups that make up the *Women's Health* Nutrition System and how they will turbocharge your weight-loss plans!

It's easy to fall into the trap of considering food your enemy. Countless diet fads over the years have demonized nearly every food group known to humankind: fat, carbs, protein, you name it. But food isn't your enemy. When eaten and enjoyed the way nature intended, food is actually your strongest weapon in your fight against fat. Not to mention the fact that it's delicious, pleasurable, nourishing, and absolutely vital to our survival. True, we actually suffer from having too much food, but the *Women's Health* Diet is about leveraging it to your advantage.

Several years ago, *Women's Health* and *Men's Health* editorial director David Zinczenko wrote the groundbreaking books *The Abs Diet* and *The Abs Diet for Women*, in which he listed a dozen critical food groups that play a role in boosting metabolism. The *Women's Health* Nutrition System simplifies that concept. By focusing on just eight food types, you'll get lean—fast—which is why we grouped them into a simple acronym for you to remember: FAST & LEAN. Everything you'll find on this list is prime body-sculpting sustenance. Anything you eat that doesn't fall into one of these categories, on the other hand, probably isn't good for you. To enhance muscle (remember, muscle is your BFF who wants to make you look fab!) and burn fat, just hit the suggested serving scores. You'll fuel your body with all the nutrients it needs, and you'll crowd out the bad foods in the process.

The Superfood Daily Cheat Sheet
Eat from this list and get lean, fast!

Fiber-rich grains .... 2–4 servings
Avocados, oils, and other healthy fats .... 1–2 servings
Spinach, leafy greens, and other vegetables .... At least 3 servings
Turkey and other lean meats................................ 2 or more servings
&
Legumes... At least 1 serving
Eggs and dairy .... 2–4 servings
Apples and other fruits .... 3 or more servings
Nuts and seeds .... At least 1 serving

The *Women's Health* FAST & LEAN Superfoods

These food groups have been specifically selected for their fat-fighting properties. Here's some of the science behind their magic.

Fiber-Rich Grains

The Highlights

Do you react to carbs the way citizens of Tokyo react to Godzilla? Relax! There's nothing inherently wrong with carbohydrates, unless food scientists get ahold of them and turn them bright orange, electric lavender, or fluorescent green. Healthy carbs made from whole grains can and should be a staple of your daily diet. They provide energy and help facilitate the muscle-building process. Whole-grain breads, pastas, and brown rice are obvious choices. But don't be afraid to branch out: Quinoa and oats are packed with fiber and are so protein-rich that they practically count as meat!

The Sciencey Stuff

Researchers at Penn State University compared those who ate whole grains to those who ate refined grains and found that whole-grain eaters lost 2.4 times more belly fat than those who ate refined grains. The high fiber helps, but these results go beyond simple satiety. Whole grains more favorably affect blood-glucose levels, which means they don't cause wild swings in blood sugar and ratchet up cravings after you eat them. Plus, the antioxidants in whole grains help control inflammation and insulin (the hormone that tells your body to store fat).

YOUR GOAL: 2–4 servings per day, aiming to eat at least 1 serving both before and after your workouts

CAVEAT: When it comes to carbs, food manufacturers love to mess with our heads. They refine our wheat, rice, and other grains, stripping out all the vitamins, minerals, and fiber found in the bran (the outside of the grain) and the germ (the very center) and leaving the nutritionally dead endosperm, which they then spray with chemical facsimiles of nutrients and call "enriched." (To get an idea of what this looks like, think of a kernel of corn. The skin on the outside is the bran, and the little tiny seed in the middle is the germ. Everything else is the endosperm.) So when you see "multigrain" or "wheat" on the label of a loaf of bread or even cereal, you probably think, "Ah, the healthy stuff!" But read the nutrition label. Often "multigrain" just means more than one grain has had the nutritional life beaten out of it and then added to the food. And as we mentioned earlier, "wheat" bread is often just refined white bread that's been dyed with molasses to look healthier. Always look on the label, and always look for "whole grain." If you see the word "refined," don't be refined at all—toss it and run.

Avocados, oils, and other healthy fats

The Highlights

Here's a nutritional secret worth remembering: Eating fat won't make you fat any more than eating money will make you rich. Indeed, the right kinds of fats can actually make you slimmer. Your body is designed to burn fat for energy. So by timing your fat intake, you'll not only trigger weight loss, you'll also fuel your workouts more effectively—and see even greater gains in the gym.

The Sciency Stuff

The two fats we want you to concentrate on are monounsaturated fats (MUFAs), the healthy oils found in olives, nuts, seeds, avocado, açai, and even chocolate; and omega-3 fatty acids, which are found in cold-water fish, grass-fed meats, nuts, seeds, and some fruits. These fats can lower your risk of heart disease, protect cells from damage, help encourage muscle growth, and increase the amounts of valuable nutrients available from other foods. But more shockingly, scientists in Italy found that people who eat diets with higher amounts of these fats actually burn more blubber during exercise. That's right: MUFAs and omega-3s are actually fat-burning fats!

But that's not the only way dietary fat helps you get rid of body fat. In a study in the *International Journal of Obesity*, researchers at Brigham and Women's Hospital, in Boston, put 101 overweight people on either a low-fat diet or a moderate-fat diet and followed them for 18 months. Both groups lost weight, but only the moderate-fat-diet group lost an average of 9 pounds per person and kept it off after a year. The reason: Fat consumption helps boost levels of a hormone called leptin, the "satiation hormone" that tells you when you're full.

YOUR GOAL: 1–2 servings per day. That might include some guacamole, some pasta with olive oil, some salad dressing. Note: You'll also be getting healthy monounsaturated fats from nuts (you'll read more about them in a moment). While you want to eat plenty of those, make sure you're also getting enough healthy fats from the above sources as well.

> **HOT TIP #89**
>
> **De-Stress With Sex.** In a study of people engaged in public speaking, those who had intercourse in the weeks prior had less severed spikes in blood pressure. Flying solo gave only half the benefits.

Spinach, leafy greens, and other vegetables

The Highlights

If there's one food off the FAST & LEAN list that has almost unlimited benefits, it's leafy green vegetables. Packed with supernutrients that can improve heart health, elevate your mood, burn off calories, and do everything from protecting your eyes to boosting your sexual health and pleasure, leafy green vegetables are the best nutritional bargain in the universe. Eat them, wherever and whenever you see them.

The Sciency Stuff

The caloric value of most vegetables is so low that the simple process of eating and digesting greens burns as many calories as what's contained in the food. Need more proof? Researchers in New York surveyed more than 2,000 dieters, and those who were most successful, felt the fullest, and lost the most weight ate at least 4 servings of vegetables per day. Plus, vegetables, especially leafy green ones like spinach and brussels sprouts, are packed with folate. As you read earlier, folate, a B vitamin, is the holy grail of nutrients. Scientists believe that the best way to tell if you're eating a healthy diet is to measure your levels of this nutrient. Folate—which, by the way, is harder and harder for Americans to come by as we move away from vegetables and toward more packaged and processed foods—has been shown to fight depression and

> **HOT TIP #90**
>
> **Go Yellow.** Yellow split peas are not only higher in protein (16 grams per cup) than green split peas, but studies show that protein might reduce blood pressure. So make a big pot of yellow pea soup.

weight gain. Indeed, in one study, dieters with the highest levels of folate lost 8.5 times as much weight as those with the lowest levels.

YOUR GOAL: At least 3 servings of vegetables each day, including fresh and frozen varieties. (But we'd prefer you eat more—vegetables are like a "get out of the hospital free" card, so eat as many of them as you can.) The easiest way to hit this number? Have a salad before your entrée as often as possible. Not only do you boost your folate, you'll slow digestion and feel satisfied for hours longer.

Turkey and other lean meats

The Highlights

Protein is the basic building block of the entire human body, and meat and eggs are the best source of it. Eating more protein is a key component of building muscle and is also your best friend in terms of dramatic body transformation and overall health. Protein does everything from giving you enviable muscle tone to trimming inches from your waist. That's because your body burns a lot of calories when it's digesting protein—about 25 calories for every 100 calories you eat (compared with only 10 to 15 calories for fats and carbs). That's called the thermic effect of eating, and it's how up to 30 percent of our calories get used up. So the more protein you eat, the more calories you burn!

The Sciency Stuff

Protein is made of amino acids, which can be split into two types: essential and nonessential. The best forms of protein include all nine essential amino acids that your body can't naturally produce. Based on this, ideal sources include poultry, pork, lean beef, fish, dairy, eggs, nuts, and oats. Other sources, such as beans, seeds, and cornmeal, provide a shot of protein, but the amount of essential amino acids in these foods falls slightly below your body's needs. Foods like bread, rice, pasta, and potatoes contain protein, but they don't contain the essential amino acids and thus are incomplete sources. A diet that primarily consists of proteins from complete sources will provide the best results.

YOUR GOAL: 2 servings per day, especially during breakfast. Be sure to eat something from this category (or from the protein-rich eggs and dairy category) as part of your preworkout and postworkout meals.

Legumes

The Highlights

What, exactly, is a legume? It's anything that grows inside a pod, such as beans, lentils, peas, edamame, peanuts, and those clones from *Invasion of the Body Snatchers.* With the exception of that last entry, legumes are basically little weight-loss pills. Every time you pop one, you're getting closer to your goal. Try to think of them that way and you'll find yourself noshing pea soup, grabbing some bean dip, buying bean burritos, or spreading peanut butter on everything.

The Sciency Stuff

One study found that people who eat ¾ cup of beans daily weigh 6.6 pounds less than those who don't eat beans, even though the bean eaters consumed 199 more calories per day. (See? Eat more, weigh less.) Another study, in the *Journal of the American College of Nutrition,* discovered that people who eat beans each day have a smaller waist size and lower blood pressure. And while too much soy isn't a good idea, especially for the guy in your life—soy contains naturally occurring chemicals that mimic estrogen and lower testosterone—edamame, with its fiber and protein, is still a smart snack choice.

YOUR GOAL: At least 1 serving a day. And remember: Legumes are weight-loss pills, with absolutely no nutritional downside. The more you can eat, the more fat you will lose and the more muscle you will build.

Eggs and dairy

The Highlights

Eggs are the most nutrient-dense food known to humans. A study published in the *International Journal of Obesity* found that dieters who ate a breakfast of eggs (yolk and all) instead of a bagel for 5 weeks lost 65 percent more weight—with no effect on their cholesterol or triglycerides. (That's right, eggs may be high in dietary cholesterol, but they won't raise *your* cholesterol—a common misconception.)

Milk, meanwhile, really does do a body good . . . and so do cheese, yogurt, and even ice cream. Most people know that the calcium in dairy strengthens your bones, but the list of other benefits is longer than the wine menu at a snooty French restaurant. Something as simple as drinking a glass of milk per day can help stave off a heart attack and stroke. In one study, British researchers found that subjects who drank milk at least once per day had a 16 percent decrease in heart disease risk and were 20 percent less likely to suffer from a stroke. The calcium in dairy lowers your blood pressure and creates a healthier environment for your heart. Another study, at Harvard Medical School, found that people

> **HOT TIP #91**
>
> **Go Low Fat For Love.** Switching from super-fatty to lean meats can lift your libido and increase your stamina in the sack.

THE **Women'sHealth** DIET

who ate three servings of dairy foods daily were 60 percent less likely
to be overweight than people who consumed less.

The Sciency Stuff

According to a report in the *Archives of Internal Medicine,* experts
believe that up to 77 percent of Americans are vitamin D deficient.
Vitamin D is important because a deficiency can make it harder for
you to lose weight. So drink your milk, and don't be afraid to reach
for 2 percent or even whole milk. The smoother, tastier versions
not only suppresses your appetite, but are also healthy for you. A
major review published in the *American Journal of Clinical Nutrition* found no association between the saturated fat in whole milk
and clogged coronary arteries. And there's no need to sweat the
calories: The difference between a serving of whole and low-fat
milk is a paltry 20 calories. Researchers in Sweden even found that
conjugated linoleic acids (CLA), which are found in dairy and beef
fat, can decrease waist size. The study followed 25 subjects either
taking or not taking CLA supplements for 4 weeks, and at the end,
the CLA-supplemented group had significantly smaller bellies.
(Treat yourself right: Get grass-fed beef and milk whenever possible. Grass-fed beef contains 60 percent more omega-3s, 200 percent more vitamin E, and two to three
times as much CLA.)

And while you're seeking out more
dairy, focus on yogurt. A University of
Tennessee study found that people who
added three servings of yogurt a day to
their diets lost 81 percent more belly fat
over 12 weeks than those who didn't eat
yogurt. While calcium played a role, a
study in the journal *Molecular Systems
Biology* found that yogurt-based bacteria

HOT TIP #92

**Feed Your Hunger,
Look Younger.**
People who
reported having
sex 4 times a week
looked ten years
younger than they
actually are,
according to a
10-year study of
3,500 adults.

can actually prevent the body from absorbing fat. Try Horizon brand—it contains the same bacteria used in the study.

YOUR GOAL: 2–4 servings per day. Be sure to eat something from this category (or from the protein-rich lean meats, legumes, or nuts categories) as part of your preworkout and postworkout meals. Eat eggs for breakfast regularly; munch on cheese at lunchtime; squeeze a yogurt in as a snack whenever you can.

The big question for yogurt: Whole fat, low fat, or fat free? These days, you're much more likely to find low-fat varieties at the grocery store. But in most cases, there's no reason not to go with whole fat. Plenty of evidence shows that fat helps quench your appetite and results in your eating fewer calories during the rest of the day. But fat does something else: It prevents the need for added sugars. For example, here's a breakdown (per 8 ounces) of three types of plain yogurt, from the USDA National Nutrient Database:

	PLAIN, WHOLE MILK	PLAIN, LOW FAT	PLAIN, FAT FREE
SUGAR (GRAMS)	10.58	17.25	17.43
CALORIES	138	143	127

By far, the smartest choice here is whole-milk yogurt. It has 40 percent less sugar and a mere 11 more calories than the skim-milk yogurt, and it actually has fewer calories than low-fat yogurt. And this is only comparing the most innocent of yogurts, the plain variety. Once you start to add fruit flavorings, many low-fat and fat-free (skim) yogurts can approach 30 grams of sugar per 8-ounce serving. Yoplait Original 99% Fat Free Strawberry, for example, delivers 27 grams of sugar per serving—more than a Kit Kat bar!

Apples and other fruits

The Highlights

As a good rule of thumb, the more colorful your diet, the healthier you're probably eating. That's because color equals nutrients. And the easiest (and tastiest) way to get color into your diet is to eat a variety of fruits—red apples, yellow pineapples, green kiwis, orange, um, oranges. Different colors represent different nutrients, so the wider the variety, the better.

The Sciency Stuff

Fruits contain natural sugars that, when broken down by your body, are synthesized in your liver. This may sound like technical nonsense, but it's an important benefit for your waistline. Because the sugar is processed in your liver, it doesn't spike your insulin levels, meaning you're less likely to store this energy as fat. Select any of your favorite fruits—either fresh or frozen—and use them (paired with protein) as a daily snack or as an energy boost before or after your workout.

YOUR GOAL: 3 or more servings each day, including fresh, frozen, and dried fruit. This is not hard. Have some raisin bran, eat an apple, and grab a couple of pieces of pineapple off the salad bar. You're done.

Nuts and seeds

The Highlights

Hunger-quenching fiber. Muscle-boosting protein. Disease-fighting vitamins. Heart-healthy, stomach-satisfying monounsaturated fats. Which should you eat? Mix and match them: Walnuts are higher in omega-3 fatty acids than even salmon; hazelnuts boast the muscle-building amino acid arginine; pecans have the highest antioxidant count of any nut; almonds are nature's version of vitamin E supplements. Pumpkin seeds and sunflower seeds, as well as others, are packed with vitamin E and healthy fats, too.

The Sciency Stuff

When researchers at Purdue University had people eat 2 ounces of almonds (about 48) a day for 23 weeks, they found that not only did the subjects not gain weight but they also decreased their caloric intake from other unhealthy food sources and improved their cholesterol levels. And researchers from Georgia Southern University found that eating a high-protein, high-fat snack, such as almonds, increases your resting calorie burn for up to 3.5 hours. Another study found that people who ate pistachios for 3 months lost an average of 10 to 12 pounds. According to a study in the *Journal of Nutrition*, you can snack on nuts without worrying about accumulating extra pounds, because the body doesn't absorb all the fat in nuts.

YOUR GOAL: At least 1 serving a day

The *Women's Health* Nutrition System in Action

Here's a quick look at your daily diet plan. (Yep, it's a lot of food!)

BREAKFAST(S)

FOCUS ON: Dairy, eggs, whole grains, fiber, eating a lot of calories

When you shift calorie intake to the morning, you lose weight and keep it off. So eat a large portion of your daily calories—30 to 35 percent of your total intake—in the morning. If you usually skip breakfast, ease into it with something very light, like a slice of cheese or a glass of milk with whole-wheat toast. Just make sure you start your day with some protein and some carbohydrates. The protein and carbs in dairy slow muscle protein breakdown, which promotes muscle growth and fat loss, lessen muscle damage, and reduce inflammation. And, according to Australian scientists, drinking milk for breakfast limits afternoon and nighttime binges.

HOT TIP #93

See better in color. Heirloom carrots in red, purple, and yellow pack more sight-protecting nutrients than the everyday orange variety.

You'll discover that you actually eat fewer calories throughout the day if you eat more of them in the morning, and you gain less weight simply by eating two breakfasts every day. That's right—you'll lose weight if you eat more.

So, why the "(s)"? Because if you don't have the time or appetite to eat a big meal first thing in the morning, you still want to shift as many of your calories to the first third of the day as possible. So if all you can manage is a glass of milk when you first get up, give your brain and your body a boost an hour later by eating a protein-packed meal that includes vegetables or fruit for mood-boosting brainpower. Have walnut-flax oatmeal with some yogurt and blueberries for a shot of omega-3s and brain-busting antioxidants. If you're about to hit the gym, a protein-packed smoothie combining fruits and a scoop of whey powder might be your best bet.

LUNCH

FOCUS ON: Vegetables, beans, fruits, nuts, whole grains, and packing in as much nutrition as possible

Lunch is the defining moment of your nutritional day. Breakfast is all about eating as much as you can; by dinner the day's shot. It's at lunchtime when everything comes together. It's also the meal where we have the least control over our food intake, especially at work. So be smart: Aim for a lunch that has at least three representatives from the fruit, vegetable, or legume category—they're mainly water, fiber, and vitamins, so they will keep you hydrated and full with healthy calories. Salads and soups are the easy choices here. Then add in some combination of quality proteins, healthy fats, dairy, nuts, and whole grains.

DINNER

FOCUS ON: Leafy greens and other vegetables, lean meats, fish, beans, and legumes

Studies show that if you start your dinner with a small side salad dressed in olive oil and vinegar or with steamed folate-rich vegetables like kale, spinach, collard greens, or Swiss chard, you'll decrease your overall food intake by 12 percent while taking in satiating fiber and disease-fighting nutrients. Plus, folate-rich greens will give you a mood boost. Got that? Either eat a salad before dinner or put vegetables on your plate and eat those first. Then you can move on to the main course: lean meats, whole grains, and the like. Twice a week, eat fish, which is rich in omega-3s. Fish will lower your risk of heart disease, protect your cells from damage, and increase the amount of valuable nutrients available from other foods.

SNACKS

FOCUS ON: Dairy, protein, fiber-rich grains, fruit, nuts, beans, and legumes

You can't lose weight and keep it off unless you snack! In fact, studies show that people who avoid eating between meals may end up consuming more calories overall, mostly because hungry people make bad food choices. Think protein, think fat, think calcium—your snacks are where you should try to squeeze in extra servings of dairy. Choose plain yogurt and blueberries, red bell pepper slices and cottage cheese, whole-grain cereal and milk, apples and cheese, guacamole and tortilla chips, and walnuts and raspberries.

PREWORKOUT AND POSTWORKOUT FOODS

FOCUS ON: Dairy, lean meats, grains, nuts, and eating before and immediately after exercise

Do you have to work out? No. Then again, do you have to save for retirement? No. Do you have to check the tires on your car for safety? No. Do you have to spend time with your in-laws? No. You don't have to do anything if you don't want to. Go lie down on the couch, order a pizza, and keep up with the Kardashians if you want.

But you're a grown-up. You understand that choices have consequences. You realize that investing today—in your body, in your financial future, in your family—will pay off later. So we've created an exercise program that will help you see a lifetime of gains and begin paying off immediately— and probably a lot better than your 401(k) does. You'll read about it later.

That said, actually going to the gym is only part of the strategy. If you want to see the most dramatic changes to your body, it's important that you time your meals and snacks around your workouts. This simple trick will allow you to eat more calories to fuel muscle growth without gaining excess fat.

HOT TIP #94

Step on the scale. Do it just after you've gone to the bathroom but before you eat breakfast. Repeat every Friday. People who weigh themselves regularly are less likely to gain weight.

PREWORKOUT: When you eat before a workout, those calories go toward fueling your body to work optimally during your time in the gym—plus you'll improve your mood and give yourself the burst of energy you need to motivate yourself to exercise. Dutch and British researchers found that eating before your workout speeds muscle growth by blunting your body's receptivity to cortisol, a fat-

The *Women's Health* Diet Shopping List

FIBER-RICH GRAINS
Fresh or dried pasta, instant oatmeal (no salt or sugar added), long-grain rice (brown rice, wild rice), oats, quinoa, whole-grain bread, whole-grain cereal, whole-wheat English muffins, whole-wheat pita chips, whole-wheat flour tortilla

AVOCADOS, OILS, AND OTHER HEALTHY FATS
Avocados, canola oil, grapeseed oil, olive oil, olives, safflower oil, sesame oil

SPINACH, LEAFY GREENS, AND OTHER VEGETABLES
Fresh: Artichokes, asparagus, beets, bell peppers, bok choy, broccoli, cabbage, carrots, cauliflower, celery, collard greens, cucumbers, eggplant, garlic, green beans, kale, leeks, mushrooms, onions, peas, radishes, red-leaf lettuce, romaine lettuce, scallions, spinach, sprouts, Swiss chard, tomatoes, watercress
Frozen: Broccoli florets, peas

TURKEY AND OTHER LEAN MEATS
Buffalo, casein protein powder, chicken, cod, crab, flounder, ground grass-fed beef (15 percent fat or less), grouper, halibut, lobster, mahimahi, orange roughy, pork, salmon, scallops, sea bass, shrimp, sirloin steak, tilapia, top round, trout, tuna, turkey, turkey sausage, whey protein powder

LEGUMES
Black beans, black-eyed peas, edamame, kidney beans, navy beans, pinto beans, red lentils
Spreads: Black-bean dip, hummus, peanut butter

EGGS AND DAIRY
Cheddar cheese, chocolate milk, cottage cheese, omega-3 eggs, feta cheese, goat cheese, ice cream, mozzarella cheese, string-cheese sticks, whole-milk yogurt, whole milk or 1 to 2 percent milk

APPLES AND OTHER FRUITS
Fresh: Bananas, cantaloupe, carrots, grapes, lemons, limes, mangoes, melons, oranges, peaches, pears, pineapples
Frozen: Blueberries, raspberries, strawberries
Dried: Apricots, prunes, raisins

NUTS AND SEEDS
Almonds, cashews, ground flaxseeds, sesame seeds, sunflower seeds, walnuts
Spreads: Almond butter, cashew butter (no salt or sugar added)

SEASONINGS
Use these to add rich flavors to your meals: Basil, cayenne, chili powder, cider vinegar, cilantro, cinnamon, cumin, curry powder, low-sodium soy sauce, mint, parsley, paprika, red-pepper flakes, red wine vinegar, white wine vinegar

storing stress hormone. That speeds fat loss during your workout and for an additional 24 hours, according to scientists at Syracuse University. Just make sure to include a balance of protein and carbohydrates. Eat one serving of carbohydrates with one serving of protein around 30 minutes before your workout. Down a protein shake. People who eat a protein-and-carbohydrate-rich meal before and after their workouts build TWICE as much lean muscle as those who wait at least 5 hours to eat.

POSTWORKOUT: After your workout, consuming protein helps your body recover by providing a fresh infusion of amino acids to repair and build muscle. And carbohydrates will raise your insulin levels, which slows protein breakdown and speeds muscle growth after your workout. Eat one serving of carbohydrates with one serving of protein 30 minutes after working out. A bonus: After you lift weights, your body's fat storage pathways are shut off while your fat-burning mechanisms are turned on. So if you like the occasional cookie or cupcake, consider this the Twinkie Hour. You won't use your stored protein for energy; you'll rely instead on the carbs to replenish you. And the food you eat will not only help you reveal a sexy midsection but will also boost your fat-burning lean muscle. (Don't do this every day, okay? Added sugar is never a good habit to get into.)

> **HOT TIP #95**
>
> **Eating for two?**
> In a study of couples undergoing fertility treatments, women whose meals were packed with fish, legumes and vegetable oils were 40 percent more likely to conceive.

If, like a lot of people, you work out at lunchtime, eat one of your two snacks about 30 minutes before you work out and go directly from the gym to the lunchroom. Exercise after work? Grab a snack as you're leaving the job, then eat dinner right after the gym. Work out in the mornings? Eat a light breakfast when you get up, then have something more substantial after you exercise.

Sample *Women's Health* Diet 5-Day Meal Plan

We'd love you to work out three times a week, preferably around lunchtime. But maybe your life doesn't run that way. Maybe you need to get up early to exercise, or you can't hit the gym until the workday is through, or circumstances have conspired to make gym time a no-go for the next couple of days. Not a problem—again, the *Women's Health* Nutrition System is all about maximum flexibility for maximum muscle gain (and maximum fat burn). Just remember three rules:

• Always eat breakfast.

• Always eat a little something before you work out.

• Always eat a lot of something after you work out.

Wouldn't it be awesome if your boss were as easygoing as this?

Day One (workout day)

BREAKFAST: Walnut-flax oatmeal and milk

Oatmeal with milk, chopped walnuts, ground flax, bananas, and a sprinkle of cinnamon. The milk provides an instant surge of protein; the oats keep your blood sugar in check, which regulates future cravings; the cinnamon reduces inflammation; the walnuts and flax add omega-3s and satiating healthy fat; and the bananas add heart-healthy potassium. Choose oatmeal in the form of whole oats and nothing else, such as Old Fashioned Quaker Oats.

SNACK: Protein smoothie

Chocolate whey protein powder, milk, strawberries, and bananas. The ultimate cocktail designed to have you ready for the gym. Whey is a fast-digesting protein that will prevent any stomach discomfort during exercise, while the milk, strawberries, and bananas provide the electrolyte balance that's optimal for hydration, muscle growth, and recovery.

(WORKOUT)

LUNCH: Black-bean sandwich (black-bean dip, olives, scallion greens, sprouts, tomatoes, and lettuce on 100 percent whole-wheat bread)

The black-bean dip provides mood-boosting fiber, heart-healthy fats, and quality protein. The vegetables provide cancer-fighting antioxidants, bone-mass-boosting vitamin K, cholesterol-lowering selenium, free-radical-fighting vitamin C, and blood-pressure-lowering potassium.

HOT TIP #96

Try a lusty fruit.
Lychees pack magnesium, which boosts circulation to the pelvic region.

SNACK: Hard-boiled eggs (1–2) and apple

Hard-boiled eggs are most convenient, but it's also easy to scramble a few in the a.m. and scoop them into a microwavable container. Don't sweat the fat: It's healthy and filling. The apple will provide the carbohydrates you need to refuel after your workout.

DINNER: Almond beef stir-fry over brown rice with steamed kale

Stir-fry a frozen vegetable mix of your choice in a little canola oil. Then add thinly sliced grass-fed beef, a dash of low-sodium soy sauce, and slivered almonds. Serve it over brown rice with a side of steamed kale. Starting your dinner with low-calorie, high-fiber vegetables can decrease your overall food intake by 12 percent. The beef provides quality lean protein, plus heart-healthy omega-3s. The brown rice adds fiber, which helps stave off late-night cravings.

Day Two

BREAKFAST: Mexican scrambled egg

Scramble an egg in a little olive oil with chopped tomatoes, onions, spinach, and peppers. Top with a sprinkling of shredded Cheddar cheese.

SNACK: Whole-wheat toast with almond spread and a sliced apple

LUNCH: Ultimate tuna salad

Combine red-leaf lettuce, spinach, chunk light tuna, grape tomatoes, navy beans, Cheddar cheese, carrots, broccoli, red bell peppers, flaxseeds, and sesame seeds. Dress with olive oil and balsamic vinegar.

SNACK: Greek yogurt

Greek-style yogurt is a exerciser's dream: It's easy to carry and packed with protein. Skip yogurts with fruit and sugar; to add flavor, drop in a few berries or nuts.

DINNER: Red-lentil burritos

Sauté onions, broccoli, carrots, tomato sauce, curry powder, cumin, and chili powder. Add cooked red lentils and sun-dried tomatoes. Serve in whole-wheat tortillas with Cheddar cheese, yogurt, and cilantro. Eat with a side salad of fresh baby spinach mixed with olive oil and grated Romano cheese.

Day Three (workout day)

BREAKFAST: Whole-grain cereal, a slice of toast with almond butter and chopped dried apricots, and a glass of milk

SNACK: Cottage cheese, oatmeal, and an apple

Cottage cheese contains all the benefits of a protein shake without the blending. It's a quality source of protein that will also help you lose weight, because of its high amounts of calcium. The added oatmeal and apple will boost your energy so you can lift heavier weights and curb hunger during your workout.

(WORKOUT)

LUNCH: Indonesian chicken-salad sandwich

Mix peanut butter, a dash of water, white wine vinegar, minced garlic, and red-pepper flakes with strips of organic chicken, kale, and onion. Spread on whole-wheat bread.

SNACK: 1–2 cups (8–16 ounces) of chocolate milk

Refresh and rebuild at the same time. A study in the *Journal of the American College of Nutrition* shows that chocolate milk may be the ideal postworkout beverage for building muscle.

DINNER: Seared wild salmon with mango chutney, eggplant, and Swiss chard

Brush the salmon with a mixture of lemon juice, paprika, salt, and black pepper and then sear it in a little olive oil. On top, add a mixture of mango, bell pepper, onion, lime juice, mint, and jalapeño pepper. Eat with a side of grilled eggplant and steamed Swiss chard. (Note: We strongly recommend wild salmon over the farm-raised type, which has been fed pesticide-ridden feed and had its flesh dyed to look pink. All "Atlantic salmon" is farm-raised. Choose wild Alaskan salmon instead.)

Day Four

BREAKFAST: Berry-banana smoothie

Combine frozen blueberries, raspberries, and a banana (fresh or frozen) in a blender with yogurt. Add some 1 percent milk and peanut butter. Blend until smooth. Serve with a whole-grain English muffin with black-currant jam.

SNACK: Fried-egg-and-cheese sandwich

The eggs provide satiating protein to help you power through your day.

LUNCH: Free-range chicken salad

Combine free-range organic chicken, spinach, apples, and almonds and mix with a bit of yogurt, Dijon mustard, and celery.

SNACK: Banana and peanut butter

DINNER: Buffalo burger (no bun) topped with baked and mashed garnet yams, sautéed onions, and roasted red peppers. Serve with a side of steamed spinach.

Day Five (workout day)

BREAKFAST: Spinach omelet with yogurt and blueberries

Chop a bunch of spinach, reserving a handful, and sauté it in a little olive oil. Stir together one egg and the remaining chopped spinach, pour it over the sautéed spinach, and cook until the egg is set. The yogurt provides probiotics, which support weight loss, digestion, and healthy immune functioning. The blueberries add antioxidants, which studies suggest can help prevent cancer, diabetes, and age-related memory loss.

SNACK: Berry smoothie with whey protein

This milk-derived product continues to rule the gym. Mix it with milk instead of water if you want a bit more protein. The added fruit not only improves taste but also offers sustained energy.

(WORKOUT)

LUNCH: Split-pea soup with a baby spinach salad

SNACK: Chicken, turkey, or tuna wrap

Toss one of these standbys in a whole-wheat wrap and top it with lettuce and tomatoes for the ultimate postworkout meal.

DINNER: Almond rainbow trout with watercress and collard greens

Cook farm-raised rainbow trout in almond oil with sliced raw almonds. Top with cider vinegar and watercress. Serve with a side of collard greens sautéed in olive oil and garlic. Add a serving of ice cream for dessert, which provides a small dose of sugar that fuels muscle growth.

24 SMART FOOD FIXES THAT WILL SMOOTH OVER EVERYTHING FROM BIG-MEETING JITTERS TO BIG-DATE ANGST

You're smart. You're confident. You've got an opinion and you know how to use it. And when it comes to getting things done, Gaza peace negotiators could learn a thing or two from you.

In other words, why in the world would you ever need help with anything? The truth is, even the most pulled-together of us, the ones who seem to have an ironclad grip on life, need a little backup sometimes. Especially when you're thrown a wild pitch. Like when PMS threatens to ruin your day off, or you're suddenly facing a make-or-break career moment, or you're planning a last-minute beach vacation and want to shed a few pounds.

True, nowadays there's an app to bail you out of almost any situation. But sometimes the easiest solution isn't one you download. It's one you simply down. As in food. Because, even though you might consider food your adversary (we're talking to you, french fries), if you use it right, it can be your most powerful ally. Let these foods help you out of a jam when . . .

HOT TIP #97

Wake up to water. Drink at least 16 ounces of chilled H20 as soon as you rise. German scientists found this boosts metabolism by 24 percent for 90 minutes afterward. (A smaller amount of water had no effect.) A general rule of thumb: Guzzle at least a gallon of water a day.

YOU'VE GOT A BIG DAY AT WORK
EGGS OVER EASY WITH A SIDE OF BACON OR HAM

The protein in this power meal will keep you feeling full throughout the morning. A University of Illinois study reports that people who eat more protein and less carbs at each meal find it easier to stick to a diet than those who eat more carbs and less protein. Protein is satiating and may also boost calorie burn, the study's authors say. Plus, when you digest eggs, protein fragments are produced that can prevent your blood vessels from narrowing, which may help keep your blood pressure from rising. In fact, Canadian scientists found in a lab study that the hotter the eggs, the more potent the proteins. And frying eggs sends their temperature soaring.

YOU FORGET TO PACK A TOOTHBRUSH

MONTEREY JACK

Researchers found that eating less than one-quarter of an ounce of jack, Cheddar, Gouda, or mozzarella cheese will boost pH levels to protect your pearly whites from cavities.

YOU'RE CAUGHT IN STOP-AND-GO TRAFFIC

SUGAR-FREE CHEWING GUM

In a British study, people who chewed gum while taking math, memory, and concentration tests reported an average 13 percent drop in stress. The study's authors believe that the act of chewing might lead to subconscious associations with positive social settings (like mealtimes), which may reduce tension. (Just don't actually swallow it, okay?) Sugar-free gum has the additional benefit of knocking off bacteria, which can multiply in your mouth when you're stressed or dehydrated.

YOU LOOK IN THE MIRROR AND THINK,
"THAT LAUGH LINE WASN'T THERE YESTERDAY, WAS IT?"

GUACAMOLE

A study in the *Journal of the American College of Nutrition* found that people with a high intake of olive oil showed fewer wrinkles than those with a high intake of butter. The reason: monounsaturated fats, which are found in abundance in olive oil. So drizzle some olive oil on your salad, and if that's not convenient, grab a side of guacamole; avocados have the same monounsaturated fats as olive oil, plus plenty of fiber and healthy B vitamins.

YOU NEED TO . . . TO . . . FOCUS!

PEPPERMINT TEA

Researchers in Cincinnati found that periodic whiffs of peppermint increased people's concentration on and performance of tasks requiring sustained attention. (Sniff: "I can do this.") Keep a few bags of peppermint tea in your desk, and think of it as a scientific improvement over the alternative: British researchers discovered that sleepy people who downed a sugary, caffeinated drink like soda had slower reaction times and more lapses in attention after 80 minutes than those who drank a sugar-free beverage.

YOU'RE FACING AN AFTERNOON-LONG MEETING

GRILLED SALMON WITH SPINACH AND CARROTS

This meal is scientifically proven to prevent doodling and drooling—two potentially career-crushing side effects of soporific assemblies. Stay awake effortlessly by grabbing a seafaring sidekick for lunch. Salmon contains tyrosine, an amino acid that your brain uses to make dopamine and norepinephrine—neurochemicals that keep you alert. The brain-boosting omega-3s in salmon may also help tame your neurotic tendencies. (Opt for wild salmon when you can find it; it's significantly lower in persistent organic pollutants, aka POPs, that have been linked to obesity, and it's significantly higher in omega-3s.) Halibut and trout are good alternatives to salmon. And spinach provides the B vitamin folate, used by the brain to make the mood controllers serotonin, dopamine, and norepinephrine. A lack of folate has been linked to depression. Add carrots: Beta-carotene may help reduce the effects of oxidative stress on your memory.

HOT TIP #98

Zap the TV commercials. Foods advertised on television are usually loaded with sugar and fat. Research in the *Journal of the American Dietetic Association* reveals that a 2,000-calorie diet of such foods would exceed the RDA for sugar by 25 times and the RDA for fat by 20 times. Deflect those cues with dark-chocolate.

YOU FEEL THE SNIFFLES COMING ON

GINSENG

In a Canadian study, people who took 400 milligrams of ginseng extract a day had 56 percent fewer recurring colds than those who popped placebos. Studies suggest ginseng can turbocharge the activity of key immune cells. Another benefit: Ginseng might boost your brainpower. British researchers found that people on a cognitive test scored significantly better when they swallowed 200 milligrams of the extract an hour before taking it.

AND THIS . . .

KIWI, ORANGES, RED BELL PEPPERS

All three are packed with vitamin C. Studies suggest that taking at least 200 milligrams daily may help shorten the duration of your symptoms the next time you're under the weather. A medium-size red bell pepper has 152 milligrams; a kiwi, orange, mango, or cup of steamed broccoli all add more than 50 milligrams each.

YOU'VE GOT A BAD COUGH

HONEY

Penn State scientists found that honey is better at lessening cough frequency and severity than dextromethorphan, the most common active ingredient in over-the-counter cough meds.

YOU CAN'T STOP HICCUPING

SUGAR

A study published in the *New England Journal of Medicine* found that 1 teaspoon of table sugar, swallowed dry, cured hiccups in 95 percent of people—some of whom had been hiccuping for as long as 6 weeks.

IT'S T-MINUS 3 WEEKS UNTIL YOU'LL BE
LOUNGING ON A BEACH IN BELIZE

GREEN TEA

In a 2009 report from the American Society of Nutrition, scientists found that exercisers who drank green tea lost twice as much weight as those who didn't, and had the greatest declines in total abdominal fat.

YOU'VE GOT A 5K AND THE POLLEN COUNT
IS THROUGH THE ROOF

PINK GRAPEFRUIT

Pink grapefruit is rich in two compounds: lycopene, which has been shown to decrease symptoms of wheezing, asthma, and shortness of breath in people when they exercise; and beta-cryptoxanthin, which helps decrease inflammation in the joints and may improve the function of the respiratory system.

YOU JUST FINISHED AN INTENSE WORKOUT

COFFEE

University of Georgia scientists revealed that taking a caffeine supplement (equal to 2 cups of coffee) after exercise reduces muscle soreness more than pain relievers can. Caffeine blocks a chemical that activates pain receptors.

YOU JUST FINISHED AN INTENSE WORKOUT
AND NOW YOU WANT REWARD

CHOCOLATE MILK

According to Indiana University researchers, the ratio of carbs to protein in chocolate milk is ideal for muscle recovery and growth.

AUNT EDNA IS DRAGGING YOU TO THE ALL-YOU-CAN-EAT BUFFET

AN APPLE

Discipline ain't easy when second helpings are free. But in a study at Penn State, researchers found that those who ate an apple 15 minutes before lunch consumed a total of 15 percent fewer calories than those who drank apple juice, ate applesauce, or had nothing at all.

YOUR PMS THREATENS THOSE AROUND YOU

SAFFRON

A pinch of this exotic spice may help tame the monthly beast by increasing levels of the feel-good brain chemical serotonin, which can plummet before your period. In a recent study published in *BJOG*, a journal from the British Royal College of Obstetricians and Gynaecologists, women who took 15 milligrams of saffron extract in the morning and evening saw a significant dip in irritability, fatigue, and depression.

YOU FEEL LIFE HAS NO MEANING

FLAXSEED

Flax is the best-known source of alpha-linolenic acid, or ALA—a healthy fat that improves the workings of the cerebral cortex, the area of the brain that processes sensory information, including pleasure. To meet your quota, sprinkle it into smoothies or onto salads, or make it the secret ingredient in a PB & J.

> **HOT TIP #99**
>
> **Go for the D-cup.**
> A vitamin D deficiency can make it harder for you to lose weight, a University of Minnesota study reveals. Milk is your best dietary source of vitamin D. In another study, dieters who downed five servings of dairy a day lost more abdominal fat than those who had just three.

167

YOUR MEXICAN LUNCH KEEPS SENDING YOU REMINDERS

SAUERKRAUT

A study published in the *European Journal of Gastroenterology & Hepatology* found that Lactobacillus plantarum 299V, the bacteria used to ferment foods like sauerkraut, relieved gas symptoms in 33 of 40 people studied. (*Women's Health* editors read this kind of stuff all the time so you don't have to.)

YOU'RE ON A HOT DATE

SUSHI FOR DINNER AND DARK CHOCOLATE FOR DESSERT

Salmon and mackerel are high in omega-3 fatty acids that keep sex-hormone production humming along. Ginger is a natural blood thinner, so it aids overall circulation, increasing blood flow to your hot spots. As for the chocolate, according to the *Journal of the American Dietetic Association*, it contains a compound called phenylethylamine, which releases the same endorphins triggered by sex and increases the feelings of attraction between two people. Caveat: White chocolate won't do the trick. It has no cocoa solids, so it lacks the methylxanthines (caffeine and theobromine) found in dark and milk chocolate. These stimulants can make you feel more energetic and alert, and cocoa solids also hold the heart-healthy antioxidants that make darker chocolates so appealing to your cardiologist.

YOU'RE ON A HOT DATE AND YOU HAD THE GARLIC SHRIMP INSTEAD

MILK

A study from Ohio State, published in the *Journal of Food Science*, found that the combination of water, fat, and sodium caseinate in milk could help reduce concentrations of volatile compounds responsible for foul-smelling garlic breath.

YOU'RE ON A HOT DATE AND YOU WANT TO IMPRESS
WITH SOMETHING BESIDES YOUR DAZZLING SMILE
BLUEBERRIES

Researchers at Tufts University have found that blueberries and the anthocyanadins they contain may make brain cells respond better to incoming messages and might even spur the growth of new nerve cells. This may take more than just eating a dessert, though.

YOU'RE IN THE MOOD, HE'S IN THE MOOD,
AND YOU WANT TO MAKE A BABY
MILK (AGAIN!)

And not the low-fat variety. If you add one serving of full-fat dairy to your diet per day, such as whole milk on your cereal instead of skim, you can actually increase your chances of getting pregnant, according to the landmark Nurse's Health Study at Harvard University. And because the calcium in dairy fights weight gain, you're receiving another boost for conceiving: Maintaining a healthy weight ups your chances for getting pregnant.

YOU HAD SUCH AN AWESOME DAY
THAT YOU JUST CAN'T FALL ASLEEP
OATMEAL WITH BANANAS AND WALNUTS

Sleep is triggered by the hormone melatonin, but stress or excitement can disrupt melatonin's release. Bring your brain back down to earth by whipping up a bowl of oatmeal and topping it with sliced bananas and crushed walnuts, both

HOT TIP #100

Get up, stand up.
Americans sit 8 percent more than they did in 1980. Studies show that the more time you spend sitting, the greater your risk of heart attack, regardless of how fit you are. And standing for three 10-minute phone calls a day will burn an extra 33 calories. That's 2 pounds gone every year!

rich in melatonin. What won't do the trick: warm milk. Contrary to popular belief, warm milk will keep you up, not knock you out. Blame the protein in the milk, which can reduce serotonin levels and delay the onset of sleep.

YOU WANT TO PREVENT A HANGOVER

A VIRGIN SCREWDRIVER

For last call, order this start-the-day staple. Fructose, one of the sugars in orange juice, can speed the metabolism of alcohol, by as much as 25 percent. Vitamin C also helps combat binge-related cell damage.

YOU WAKE UP THE NEXT MORNING AND REALIZE
YOU FORGOT TO PREVENT THE HANGOVER

GATORADE AND TOAST WITH JAM

Your first order of business is to replace fluids and electrolytes lost to the dehydrating effect of alcohol. A sports beverage will accomplish this, while the fructose in jam helps metabolize the alcohol and the easy-to-digest toast fuels your energy stores—without taxing your stomach—so you can face the day with a smile.

Dark chocolate releases the same endorphins triggered by sex and makes you feel energetic and alert.

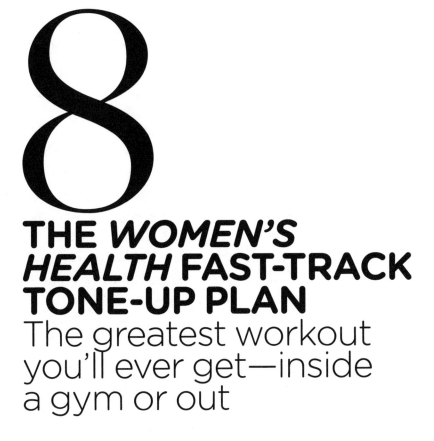

THE *WOMEN'S HEALTH* FAST-TRACK TONE-UP PLAN
The greatest workout you'll ever get—inside a gym or out

Walking into the gym and expecting a great workout is like walking into the supermarket and expecting a gourmet meal. The basic ingredients are there, but, as they say in the infomercials, results may vary. With working out, as with cooking, a little bit of smarts, dedication, creativity, and knowledge will make all the difference between perfect pasta and a gelatinous ball of mush.

In fact, your best chance at a great workout might come from avoiding the gym all together. Why? Because the run-of-the-mill fitness club already has three strikes against it.

Strike one: the trainers

There are nearly 200,000 fitness trainers at work in the United States, doing the kind of stuff that's traditionally been the province of medical professionals—giving out nutritional advice; testing our cardio, muscular, and nervous systems; and jacking up our heart rates and blood pressure with prescriptive programs. And what kind of training do these exercise experts have? In many cases, little or none. There's absolutely no governing body for trainers or set of standardized tests that they have to pass before they come to your gym or your house and start making you sweat.

Now, you might be thinking, "At my gym, they have 'certified personal trainers.'" Sure, most gyms like their trainers to be certified, but by whom? There are close to 300 US certifications available, many of them meaningless. (Want certification as a group fitness instructor from the American Fitness Professionals & Associates? Just send $370 to a P.O. box in Ship Bottom, New Jersey, and you'll get a textbook and a DVD that tells you everything you need to know. You never even have to meet with anyone. Just pass a simple test—you get to take it over and over again until you do—and you're certified!) Only two certifying bodies are really worth their salt: the National Strength and Conditioning Association (NSCA), which grants the prestigious Certified Strength and Conditioning Specialist (CSCS), and the American College of Sports Medicine (ACSM).

That said, having a personal trainer does have one solid benefit: You're paying someone for his or her time, and that alone may help you stick to a workout. Still, if you want to hire a teammate in your quest for fitness, make sure you grill him or her the way you would any potential employee. (A good starting place is our set of questions on page 192.)

Strike two: the equipment

Most gyms have rows and rows of shiny weight machines that duplicate the movements found in free-weight workouts: bench press machines, shoulder press machines, even something called a Smith machine, which duplicates a squat. But the only exercise you should be doing on machines like these? Walk-aways. Here's how you do them: You look at the machine, and then you walk away.

Two reasons: First, studies show that you simply get a better workout using free weights. Take, for instance, the leg-extension machine: University of Kentucky researchers studied 23 patients with knee pain to see which exercise made them stronger, using a simple set of stairs or using one of these machines. They found that in every measure of leg strength, simple stepups using a flight of stairs built strength more effectively. The leg-extension machine didn't make test subjects stronger at any tasks at all, except one: using the leg-extension machine. It did nothing for how test subjects functioned in the real world. Another study, in the *Journal of Strength and Conditioning Research,* found that subjects who did squats using free weights activated 43 percent more muscle than those who performed squats on the Smith machine.

Second, machines may seem safer, but they can lead to injury, because they lock our bodies into planes of movement that aren't natural. For example, when you walk or climb a set of stairs or do squats using a light weight, your thighbone rotates under your kneecap—the normal movement of your lower body. But on a leg-extension machine, your kneecap rotates instead. That puts a lot of strain on the knee ligaments and patella, the soft padding under the kneecap.

So if exercise machines are both ineffective and dangerous, why are gyms so packed with them? Simple: Because they want you to think you can't get a great workout without all that fancy equipment, so you'll have to keep coming back to the gym! The *Women's Health* Fast-Track Tone-Up Plan, on the other hand, requires only a single set of dumbbells, and you don't even need a gym. You can perform it in your living room, basement, high school auditorium, walk-in closet, cubicle, or whatever facility you might have access to.

You can, by the way, also do it at your local fitness club. (And if you do happen to swing by the gym, familiarize yourself first with our list of exercise machines you should never, ever use, on page 188.)

Strike three: the sweaty crowds

Every moment you spend standing around waiting for the bench press or a cable station is less time you spend challenging your muscles and igniting your metabolism. More sitting around means less intensity, and that undercuts your ability to make quick gains from your time in the gym. And with less time than ever to exercise, you need a workout that guarantees results, fast.

That's why *Women's Health* has designed this fat-burning, body-toning workout that uses minimum equipment and gets maximum efficiency: 10 exercises performed as a high-intensity circuit that works every muscle in your body.

But this isn't your traditional program filled with the standard 3 sets of 10 reps. Those are arbitrary goals set by some gym teacher back in sixth grade. This plan works by time—the ultimate motivator—and it allows you to challenge your body and push your fitness to new levels. Instead of worrying about a goal number of reps, each set is timed so you can push yourself to reach a new personal record each workout. This approach allows you to choose whether you want to perform more reps or add more weight, putting you in control of your goal. You'll be changing your body, strengthening your heart, and doing everything you need to look and live healthier than ever.

THE *WOMEN'S HEALTH* DIET FAST-TRACK TONE-UP PLAN

Instructions Do this circuit 3 days a week. Perform 1 set of each exercise in succession. Each set consists of doing the exercise as many times as you can in 30 seconds. Use only perfect form—it doesn't count if you cheat—and when your 30 seconds are up, give yourself 15 seconds to rest before moving on to the next exercise. Rest for 2 minutes after you've completed the entire sequence. Then repeat the whole process two more times for a total of 3 circuits per workout.

If you get tired and can't continue exercising for the entire 30 seconds, stop and rest for a few seconds and then resume performing reps until the time is up. For each exercise, you should start with a weight that you can use for 10 to 12 reps.

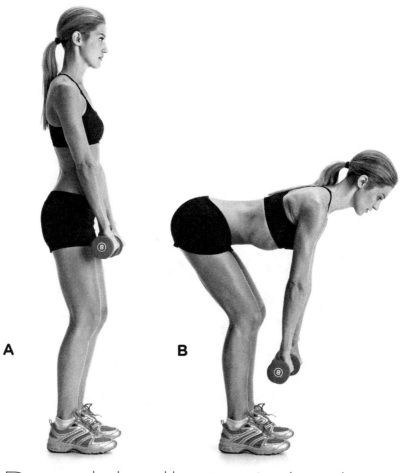

A   B

Dumbbell straight-leg deadlift

Grab a pair of dumbbells with an overhand grip and hold them in front of your thighs, arms hanging straight down. Stand with your feet hip-width apart and your knees slightly bent (A). Without changing the bend in your knees, bend at your hips, and lower your torso until it's almost parallel to the floor (B). Pause, then raise your torso back to the starting position.

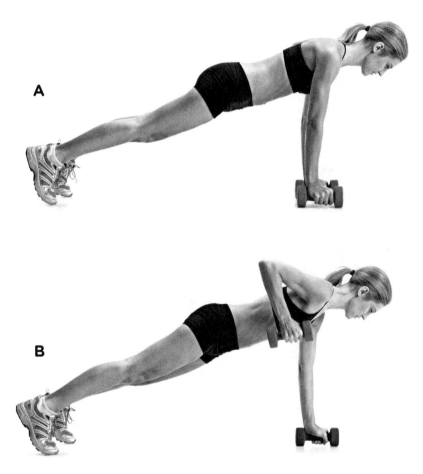

A

B

Push-up position dumbbell row

Grab a pair of hex dumbbells and assume a push-up position, with your arms straight. Your body should form a straight line from your head to your ankles (A). Keeping your core braced, balance your weight on your left arm as you row the dumbbell in your right hand up to the side of your chest, bending your arm as you pull it upward (B). Pause, then quickly lower the dumbbell. Repeat with your left arm.

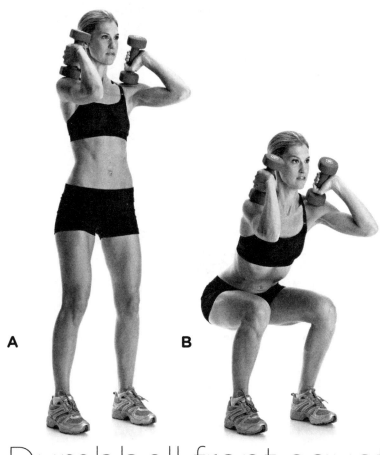

A   **B**

Dumbbell front squat

Stand and hold a pair of dumbbells so that your palms are facing
each other, and rest one of the dumbbell heads on the fleshiest part of
each shoulder (A). Keep your body as upright as you can at all times.
Brace your abs, and lower your body as far as you can by pushing your
hips back and bending your knees (B). Don't allow your elbows to drop
down as you squat. Pause, then push yourself back to the starting position.

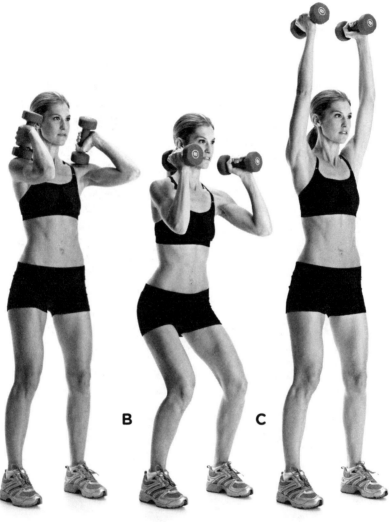

A   B   C

Dumbbell push press

Stand and hold a pair of dumbbells so that your palms are facing each other, and rest one of the dumbbell heads on the fleshiest part of each shoulder (A) or hover just above them. Keep your body upright as you bend slightly at the knees (B), then explosively push up with your legs as you press the dumbbells over your head (C). Pause, then lower the weights to the starting position.

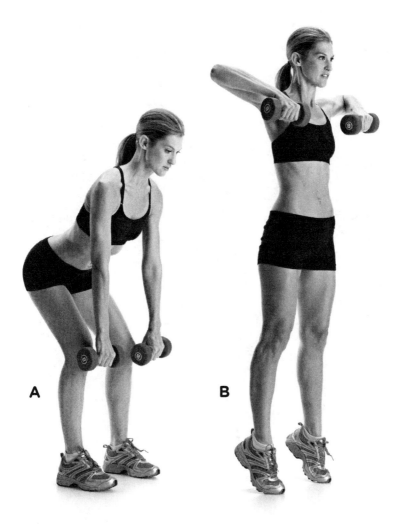

A　　　　　　　　**B**

Dumbbell hang pull

Hold a pair of dumbbells just below your knees with your palms
facing your legs, your hips pushed back, and knees slightly bent (A). Pull
both dumbbells upward as fast as you can by bending your elbows,
thrusting your hips forward, and explosively standing up. Keep the dumbbells as close to your body as possible and bring them up to shoulder
height (B). (At the top of the movement, your elbows should angle out
like you're doing the funky chicken.) Return to the starting position.

A

B

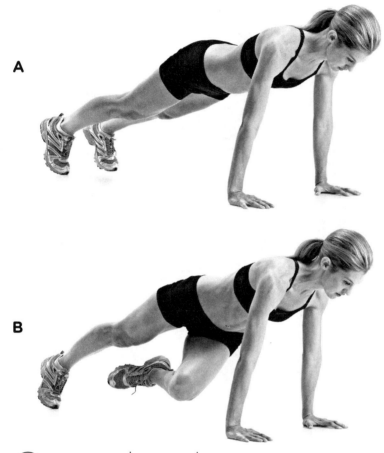

Cross-body mountain climber

Assume a push-up position with your arms completely straight. Your body should form a straight line from your head to your ankles (A). Lift your left foot off the floor, then bend your left knee and bring it up under your body, toward your right elbow, without changing the arch in your lower back (B). Lower your leg back to the starting position. Then raise your right foot off the ground and bring your right knee to your left elbow. Alternate back and forth until time is up.

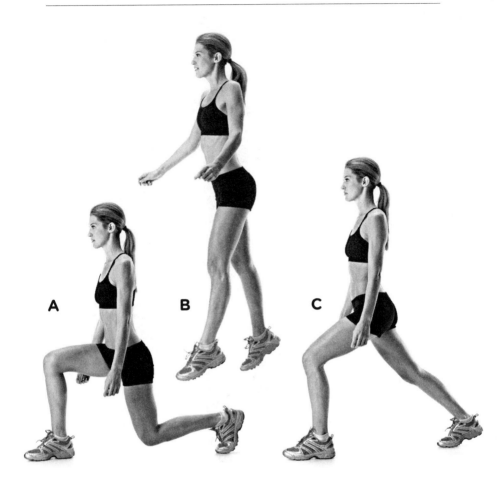

A   B   C

Alternating split jump

Stand in a staggered stance with your feet 2 to 3 feet apart, your right foot in front of your left. Keeping your torso upright, bend your legs and lower your body into a lunge position. At the bottom of the movement, your right thigh should be parallel to the ground and your left thigh should be perpendicular to the ground (A). Now jump with enough force to propel both feet off the floor (B). While you're in the air, scissor-kick your legs so you land with your left leg forward and right leg behind you (C). Repeat, alternating your forward leg for the duration of the set.

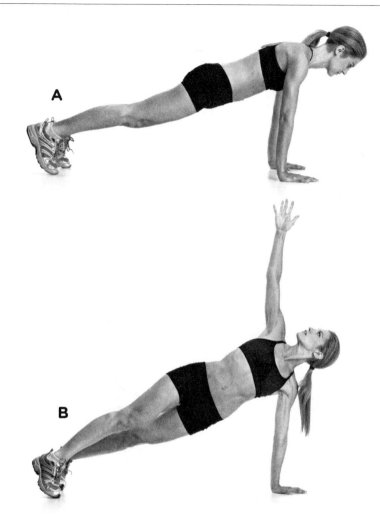

A

B

T-Stabilizer

Assume a push-up position. Your body should form a straight line from your head to your ankles (A). Keeping your arms straight and your body rigid, shift your weight onto your left arm and rotate your torso up and to the right until you're facing sideways (B). Pause for 3 seconds, then lower back down to the starting position. Rotate to your left. Continue to rotate back and forth for 30 seconds.

MAKE IT HARDER: Perform the move with a hex dumbbell in each hand and/or do a push-up each time you return to the starting position.

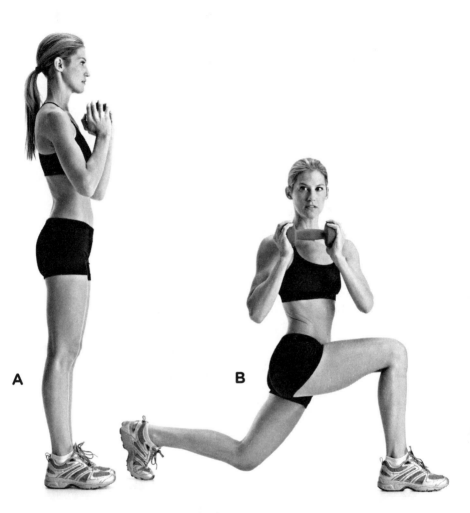

A

B

Dumbbell lunge and rotation

Grab a dumbbell and hold it by the ends just below your chin (A).
Step forward into a lunge. As you lunge, rotate your upper body
toward the same side as the leg you're using to step forward (B).
Return to the starting position and repeat on the other side. Continue
rotating to each side for the duration of the set.

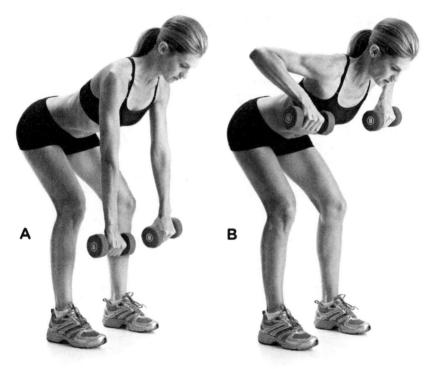

Dumbbell row

Grab a pair of dumbbells, bend at your hips (don't round your lower back), and lower your torso until it's nearly parallel to the floor. Let the dumbbells hang at arm's length (A). Without moving your torso, row the weights upward by raising your upper arms, bending your elbows, and squeezing your shoulder blades together. Keep the dumbbells close to the side of your body at the top of the movement (B). Pause, lower the dumbbells, and repeat.

The 10 Exercise Machines You Must Avoid

Think you're supposed to be lining up behind those sit-up chairs and hip-abductor contraptions? Think again. Many of the most popular machines in the gym not only train your muscles incorrectly, they put stress on your joints and can lead to injury. For this list of no-no machines, we consulted Stuart McGill, PhD, professor of spine biomechanics at the University of Waterloo, in Ontario, Canada; Nicholas DiNubile, MD, author of *FrameWork: Your 7-Step Program for Healthy Muscles, Bones, and Joints;* and trainer Vern Gambetta, author of *Athletic Development: The Art & Science of Functional Sports Conditioning.*

1. SEATED LEG EXTENSION

WHAT IT'S SUPPOSED TO DO: Train the quadriceps

WHAT IT ACTUALLY DOES: It strengthens a motion that your legs aren't designed to do and can put undue strain on the ligaments and tendons surrounding the kneecaps.

A BETTER EXERCISE: One-legged bodyweight squats. Lift one leg up and bend the opposite knee, dipping as far as you can, with control, while flexing at the hip, knee, and ankle. Use a rail for support until you develop requisite leg strength and balance. Aim for 5 to 10 reps on each leg. (If you are susceptible to knee pain, do the Bulgarian split squat instead, resting the top of one foot on a bench positioned 2 to 3 feet behind you. Descend until your thigh is parallel to the ground and then stand back up. Do 5 to 10 reps per leg.)

2.
SEATED MILITARY PRESS

WHAT IT'S SUPPOSED TO DO: Train shoulders and triceps

WHAT IT ACTUALLY DOES: Overhead pressing can put shoulder joints in vulnerable biomechanical positions. It puts undue stress on the shoulders, and the movement doesn't let you use your hips to assist your shoulders, which is the natural way to push something overhead.

A BETTER EXERCISE: Medicine-ball throws. Stand three feet from a concrete wall; bounce a rubber medicine ball off a spot on the wall 4 feet above your head, squatting to catch the ball and rising to throw it upward in one continuous motion. Aim for 15 to 20 reps. Alternative: Standing alternate dumbbell presses. As you push the right dumbbell overhead, shift the right hip forward. Switch to the left side.

3.
SEATED LAT PULLDOWN (Behind the neck)

WHAT IT'S SUPPOSED TO DO: Train lats, upper back, and biceps

WHAT IT ACTUALLY DOES: Unless you have very flexible shoulders, it's difficult to do correctly, so it can cause pinching in the shoulder joint and damage the rotator cuff.

A BETTER EXERCISE: Incline pullups. Place a bar in the squat rack at waist height, grab the bar with both hands, and hang from the bar with your feet stretched out in front of you. Keep your torso stiff and pull your chest to the bar 10 to 15 times. To make it harder, lower the bar; to make it easier, raise the bar.

4.
SEATED PEC DECK

WHAT IT'S SUPPOSED TO DO: Train chest and shoulders

WHAT IT ACTUALLY DOES: It can put the shoulder in an unstable position and place excessive stress on the shoulder joint and its connective tissue.

A BETTER EXERCISE: Incline pushups. See number 3, "Seated Lat Pulldown," but use the bar for pushups instead of pullups. Aim for 15 to 20 reps. If this is too easy, progress to regular pushups and aim for 5 to 8 reps.

5. SEATED HIP ABDUCTOR MACHINE

WHAT IT'S SUPPOSED TO DO: Train outer thighs

WHAT IT ACTUALLY DOES: Because you are seated, it trains a movement that has no functional use. If done with excessive weight and jerky technique, it can put undue pressure on the spine.

A BETTER EXERCISE: Place a heavy, short looped resistance band around your legs (at your ankles); sidestep out 20 paces and back with control. This is much harder than it sounds.

6. SEATED ROTATION MACHINE

WHAT IT'S SUPPOSED TO DO: Train abdominals and obliques

WHAT IT ACTUALLY DOES: Because the pelvis doesn't move with the chest, this exercise can put excessive twisting forces on the spine.

A BETTER EXERCISE: Do the cable wood chop. Stand with a high pulley machine on your right side. Hold the handle with both hands and straighten your arms. Pull the handles straight across your body and down in a diagonal motion, until it is outside your left knee; you should let your heels turn freely with your torso. Aim for 10 to 12 reps.

7. SEATED LEG PRESS

WHAT IT'S SUPPOSED TO DO: Train quadriceps, glutes, and hamstrings

WHAT IT ACTUALLY DOES: It often forces the spine to flex without engaging any of the necessary stabilization muscles of the hips, glutes, shoulders, and lower back.

A BETTER EXERCISE: Body-weight squats. Stand with your feet shoulder-width apart, hands straight out in front of you at shoulder level. Brace your core, then lower your body by pushing your hips back and bending your knees until your thighs are parallel to the floor or lower. Keep your weight on your heels for the entire movement. Focus on descending with control as far as you can without rounding your lower back. Aim for 15 to 20 for a set and increase sets as you develop strength.

8.
SQUATS USING SMITH MACHINE

WHAT IT'S SUPPOSED TO DO: Train chest, biceps, and legs

WHAT IT ACTUALLY DOES: The alignment of the machine—the bar is attached to a vertical sliding track—makes for linear, not natural, arched movements. This puts stress on the knees, shoulders, and lower back.

A BETTER EXERCISE: Body-weight squats (see number 7, "Seated Leg Press" for instructions.)

9.
ROMAN CHAIR BACK EXTENSION

WHAT IT'S SUPPOSED TO DO: Train spinal erectors

WHAT IT ACTUALLY DOES: Repeatedly flexing the back while it's supporting weight places pressure on the spine and increases the risk of damaging your discs.

A BETTER EXERCISE: The bird-dog. Crouch on all fours, extend your right arm forward, and extend left leg backward. Do ten 7 second reps and then switch to the opposite side.

10.
ROMAN CHAIR SIT-UP

WHAT IT'S SUPPOSED TO DO: Train abdominals and hip flexors

WHAT IT ACTUALLY DOES: The crunching motion can put undue stress on the lower back when it is in a vulnerable rounded position.

A BETTER EXERCISE: The plank. Lie face-down on the floor. Prop up on your forearms, palms down. Rise up on your toes. Keep your back flat and contract your glutes, abdominals, and lats to keep your butt from sticking up. Hold this pose for 20 to 60 seconds.

BONUS: **How to Find a Personal Trainer**

Even if you love the *Women's Health* Fast-Track Tone-Up Plan—and we know you will—sometimes hiring a trainer to put you through the paces is the extra motivation you need to help you stick to a routine. As we said earlier, just because a trainer is certified doesn't mean he or she is any good. If you really want to make sure you're hiring someone who knows what he or she is doing, you need to conduct a killer interrogation. We went to Alwyn Cosgrove, the owner of Results Fitness in Santa Clara, California, and Mike Boyle, owner of Mike Boyle Strength & Conditioning in Winchester, Massachusetts—two of the brightest fitness minds at two of the best gyms in the world. They shared exactly what they look for when they hire new staff members. Here are the questions you should ask when you go searching for a trainer.

1) DO THEY EVALUATE YOU FIRST?

A trainer can't take you to where you want to go until he or she knows where you're starting from. There are different ways that a trainer can evaluate your body, but you need to be active during the process. No trainer should ever write a program without seeing how you move and assessing your weaknesses. Remember, the benefit of having a trainer is that you receive personalized feedback designed for you.

2) HOW GOOD IS HIS OR HER PROGRAM?

You don't need an advanced degree in order to find this out. Here are three signs that your trainer has developed a good program.

1) LENGTH OF TIME. A program should consider both your short- and long-term goals. But trainers worth their salt should have a vision of how to address your flaws and design a program that lasts for a decent length of time. That doesn't mean you shouldn't see results fast. In fact, you should begin seeing changes in only a few weeks. But you want your trainer to provide a plan that goes beyond those initial changes and helps you stay healthy for good.

2) CONSISTENCY. A trainer who changes the workout every single time is not allowing you to adapt and improve. As you'll experience with the *Women's Health* Fast-

Track Tone-Up Plan, you need to have a set program that will allow your body to adapt as you become stronger and lose more body fat. It may seem beneficial to change exercises every day, but that will actually prevent you from seeing rapid changes in fat loss and muscle gain. Also, if you make changes every time, you'll never know what works.

3) PROGRESSION. Just because your program doesn't change daily doesn't mean that your trainer shouldn't eventually introduce new challenges for your body. A good workout should add in some variety 4 to 6 weeks. If added sooner, it means your trainer is guessing and doesn't have a set plan for how you can improve.

3) DO THEY KEEP GOOD RECORDS?

The best trainers learn from experience. That means every workout that has ever been performed under his or her guidance should be recorded. Your progress will be based—in part—on knowing where you started, how far you came, what worked, and what didn't. And your journey should be aided by the trainer's record of other clients who had similar situations—whether they were exercising for weight loss or training for a 5-K. If your trainer does not keep records—for you or any other client—find someone who is more organized and treats their job like a business.

4) DO THEY LOOK HOW YOU WANT TO LOOK?

It might sound superficial, but your trainer's looks do matter. Your best guarantee of results is to find a trainer who possesses a similar physique to your own, only better. That doesn't mean your trainer has to look exactly like you or

even have the same body parts. But a bodybuilder is a bodybuilder and will likely train you like you're one.

5) DO THEY CONTINUE THEIR EDUCATION?

Remember that the personal training industry is a relatively young field. And between new research and the lessons learned on the training floor, conventional wisdom can change on a yearly basis. The best trainers are the ones who are constantly learning by continuing their education. Fitness seminar attendance is one of the best ways to determine whether your trainer is staying updated on how to keep you looking good and feeling healthy. Ask any potential trainer about the last seminar he or she attended. If it's been longer than three months, consider that a red flag.

9

IF YOU'RE NOT HAVING FUN, YOU'RE DOING SOMETHING WRONG

How to adapt the *Women's Health* Fast-Track Tone-Up Plan to meet your own needs and make sure you never, ever get sore, tired, or bored!

The two of you used to be a perfect team. Together you had fun. You challenged each other, and day by day you could feel yourself growing stronger and healthier and maybe even a bit wiser, too. It felt as though you had finally found the long-term relationship that would bring you eternal bliss.

But as time passed, something changed. Once, your partner inspired an unbridled passion that brought you to new peaks of physical exultation. Now you have to drag yourself to visit, and when you arrive, you just don't feel the same pull, the same desire. You look in your partner's direction and all you can see is dull deadweight.

Well, don't worry. After a couple of years together, a lot of us start to feel that way about our exercise routines.

There are many reasons any great exercise partnership—with a gym, with a particular workout, with a treadmill— can eventually go south. And these road- blocks to fitness affect the vast majority

of us: More than 80 percent of women exercise less than two times a week, according to the Centers for Disease Control and Prevention. It's not that we're ignorant or lazy. On the contrary, we argu- ably know a lot more about, and take better care of, our bodies than our counterparts with Y chromosomes. And yet, while we may start an exercise plan with the best intentions, we often fall off the wagon. Here are the three most common reasons why:

> **HOT TIP #101**
>
> **Go loco for coco.**
> Instead of a tradi- tional sports drink, grab a coconut water for a post- workout boost. It's lower in calories and has loads of electrolytes and potassium.

1. Lack of progress

Too much work for too little reward. Lack of progress is cited in studies a lot, and there's a reason: there are so many one-size-fits- all fitness programs out there, most of which don't take nutrition into account (and nutrition is key to any weight-loss plan). Fortu- nately, the *Women's Health* Fast-Track Tone-Up Plan is a proven formula with proven results, created by our *Women's Health* fitness experts and tested by people just like you. It wasn't until we had the fitness-and-nutrition formula just right—the meal plans and the exercises and the special extras that you'll find in this chapter—that we unleashed the information in this book.

2. Lack of time

You are not a hotel heiress. You don't have endless stretches of time to spend in the gym doing every exercise on the planet. You have a job, friends, family, and an ever-growing pile of laundry that needs folding. So you need a program that is efficient, a program that will make you work hard, a program that will have you seeing results, and most of all, you need a program that's going to be fun. Some of these are inherently built into the *Women's Health* Fast-Track Tone-Up Plan. You'll be moving faster than ever—and that includes dropping fat like you've never done.

3. Lack of excitement

This one's a biggie. It's like the flat tire on a getaway road trip or the rain on your wedding day (thank you, Alanis): Unless you account for it and make a plan to avoid it, it will destroy all your best-laid plans. And here's the real bummer: The more you need to get in shape, the harder boredom fights to drag you down. No kidding. Researchers reporting in the *Journal of Nutrition Education and Behavior* found that people who are out of shape have a more diffi-cult time enjoying exercise and maintaining a positive attitude about losing weight. That causes frustration, which inevitably leads them to quit the very thing they need most.

The other problem with boredom is that even if you manage to fight back, to stick with your same old routine, you'll eventually find your fitness plan stops working as well as it used to. That's right, boredom eventually erodes exercise gains, even if you show up for every session! In fact, scientists have found that when you stick with only one type of exercise for too long, it can decrease calorie burning by up to 25 percent! It's not that the exercises you're doing stop working; it's that you simply become bored with the same old shtick, so you work out with less intensity and don't see any changes.

So what's an unmotivated, gym-weary gal supposed to do?

Sister, you came to the right place . . .

The Workout That Never Leaves You Bored

The basic *Women's Health* Fast-Track Tone-Up Plan outlined in the previous chapter is unlike any other fitness plan you've ever tried, and it's nearly—nearly—boredom-proof. By getting rid of snooze-inducing exercise clichés like doing a preset number of reps and hanging around between sets, you'll be moving your body—and seeing your body change—faster than ever. And, just in case you like as much variety in your gym as Madonna likes in her boy toys, this chapter includes a complete set of alternate exercises that you can swap in wherever, whenever.

Still, even the most intense, effective, revolutionary workout routine in the world is, in the end, a routine. And that's why the best way to stick to, and supercharge, your workout is to stop thinking that exercise has to involve, well, working out.

See, everything you do that involves a little bit of effort, a little bit of movement, and a little bit of fun can and should be considered exercise. So the sooner you start seeing "having fun" as an essential aspect of "exercising," the sooner you'll begin to burn fat and build muscle more effectively. In fact, a study in the journal *Sports Medicine* found that adding a wide range of activities of varying difficulties—including types of exercise that you enjoy—helps decrease boredom and increases your enjoyment of exercise. And when you enjoy exercise more, you're more likely to stick to your plan and reach your goals.

And we're not just talking about intense, physically challenging adventures like climbing a cliff face or surfing a tsunami. Baylor University scientists found that when you combine different forms of exercise, such as mixing high- and low-intensity activity, you experience faster improvements in strength and weight loss than you would if you went full-throttle every time. That means that if you do the high-intensity *Women's Health* Fast-Track Tone-Up Plan one day, even a relaxing walk in the woods the next day will add just as much to your overall fitness as taking up an ax and chopping down said woods. Whether it's piecing together new Ikea furniture (30 minutes of work will burn more than 140 calories!) or running around with your kids (that's another 160), you'll find that engaging in your favorite everyday activities is the best way to eliminate the boredom of exercise—and change the way you look.

Your Weekly Workout Plan

Here's what you need to remember about the *Women's Health* Fast-Track Tone-Up Plan: You should only be lifting weights 3 days per week. And each of those workouts should take 45 minutes or less. But a good workout doesn't end when you put down the weights. In fact, that's when fat burning and muscle enhancing kick into high gear.

Don't forget, after you lift weights, your metabolism stays elevated for up to another 48 hours and the micro-tears in your muscles are repairing and growing stronger. That's why after you exercise hard, your muscles feel tight and sore: You can't extend your arms, laughing hurts, and your legs feel like they were dipped in concrete. This phenomenon is called delayed onset muscle soreness, or DOMS. Normally when you're feeling a bit sore, your instinct might be to lie low and cut down on your physical activity for a day or two. Besides, you worked hard at the gym—you deserve to take it easy, right?

But restricting movement is actually the worst thing for your body. It might make sense to take a day off from strength training, but the *International Journal of Sports Medicine* found that low-intensity activity on your off days is the best way to improve recovery and increase lean muscle mass.

This is where having fun on your off day has extra benefits. Your favorite hobby or activity helps the healing process by speeding up the flow of nutrients to your muscles, which repairs your muscle tissue. That's why it's called active recovery, or active rest: because it soothes your aches and pains and prepares your body for the best possible workout the next time you lift weights. Another study in the *International Journal of Sports Medicine* found that cyclists who practiced active recovery strategies performed better on sub-

Three Steps to the Fastest Results

Don't worry, it's easier than you think!

1. Perform the *Women's Health* Fast-Track Tone-Up Plan three times a week.
2. Add 2 to 3 active recovery days per week, consisting of at least 20 minutes of super-fun activity.
3. ALWAYS have at least 1 off day when you completely relax. If you feel worn out, you can bump that up to 2 off days. Pushing your body too hard will slow you down and limit your results.

sequent training sessions than those who took a day off and performed no activity. What's more, according to a study in the journal *Medicine & Science in Sports & Exercise*, active recovery strategies also help keep your metabolism chugging along for even more-sustained fat burning. While the physical benefits are undeniable, active recovery is essential to the mental aspect of making exercise enjoyable. A study in the *British Journal of Sports Medicine* found that low-intensity exercise on off days had a positive effect on psychological recovery by removing the monotony of traditional exercise programs and helping increase relaxation.

Each week you should make these activities a built-in part of your workout, in addition to your weight training. They can be things you already love to do or an activity you've never tried before. Just don't go above 60 to 70 percent of your maximum heart rate, according to researchers, and limit your activity to 30 minutes or so. You'll quickly find that you'll not only have more energy and feel better, but you'll also be psychologically refreshed and more excited about exercise. This will help you stay consistent and reach your goals.

Here's what a typical workout week could look like:

DAY 1: *Women's Health* Fast-Track Tone-Up Plan

DAY 2: Active recovery: 20 minutes

DAY 3: *Women's Health* Fast-Track Tone-Up Plan

DAY 4: Day off

DAY 5: *Women's Health* Fast-Track Tone-Up Plan

DAY 6: Active recovery: 20 minutes

DAY 7: Day off

So what counts as an active recovery day? It can be almost any movement that gets your blood flowing. That might mean taking a walk, sweeping the floor, or running around with your kids or your dog. The intensity can vary, but as long as you're not straining your muscles with added resistance, your body will benefit.

For active recovery days, choose from the list of options below. Any of these activities count as exercise!

Exercise/Sports

Badminton	Ice Skating	Snowboarding
Basketball	Jumping rope	Soccer
Billiards	Kayaking/rowing	Softball
Bowling	Kickball	Swimming
Capoeira	Kickboxing/	Tennis
Cycling/spinning	mixed martial arts	Volleyball
Dancing	Racquetball	Walking
Frisbee	Rock climbing	Waterskiing
Golf	Rollerblading	Wii
Hiking	Running	Yoga
Horseback riding	Skiing	Zumba

Home Maintenance

Cleaning	Mowing lawn	Sweeping
Digging	Painting	Vacuuming
Gardening	Raking	
Moving furniture	Shoveling	

Home Life

Having sex	Playing with your kids	Walking the dog

So, does this mean you have to ride a Jet Ski, play tennis, make whoopee, try Pilates, learn to juggle, take up archery, mountain bike a back road, or wrestle an alligator only on "active recovery" days? No. As long as you give yourself at least one day of pure rest each week, you can do all these fun things every day if you'd like. But the prescription here is that you need to do them at least twice a week to keep your muscles healthy, your metabolism revving, and boredom at bay. Deal? Okay, let's go have some fun!

Three Ways to Customize the *Women's Health* Fast-Track Tone-Up Plan

We all hit plateaus in life. Whether you're waiting for a pay raise or trying to take your relationship to the next level, exercise is no different. Sometimes you just seem to be stuck. But it doesn't have to be that way. The exercises in the *Women's Health* Fast-Track Tone-Up Plan were carefully selected by our top fitness advisors and crafted to maximize results in the shortest time possible. But the workout is also flexible and was created to help you achieve a better body for the rest of your life. Use the following adjustments to provide a new spin to the *Women's Health* Fast-Track Tone-Up Plan, so your workout never goes stale and you continually see improvements to your body.

1: Supercharge Your Metabolism

Ready to kick up your fitness another notch? Increase the difficulty of the *Women's Health* Fast-Track Tone-Up Plan by performing each exercise for 60 seconds (instead of 30). You'll experience more of the benefits of this state-of-the-art fitness system, and take your body to the next level.

2: Fire Up Your Muscle

If you're willing to add a few more dumbbells to your workout, you can perform each exercise for the 30-second time period using the heaviest weight you can use for each exercise. So rather than just using one pair of dumbbells for the entire workout, you will build maximum strength on each lift. Select a weight that you could normally use for 8 to 10 repetitions.

3: Exercise Switch & Swap

The exercises in the *Women's Health* Fast-Track Tone-Up Plan work all of your main muscle groups from every angle while incorporating real-life movements. But your workouts aren't limited to those 10 exercises. Follow the original plan for at least 6 weeks, and after that time period, select any of the alternate moves from the list below and rotate them in your workout. Remember, you'll still perform only 10 exercises, but this will allow for more variety. You can perform 9 exercises from the original workout and just change one. Or you can change all 10. By adding these new moves, you'll literally create hundreds of different workouts that will have you seeing results after just a few weeks and still making improvements after a year. The movement patterns are similar, but the new exercises will challenge your body in a slightly different way, which will help you avoid plateaus and have you wanting to strut around in a bikini even when you're not at the beach.

Here are 10 new exercises you can use as upgrades and to switch things up.

STANDARD EXERCISE:
DUMBBELL STRAIGHT-LEG DEADLIFT
THE UPGRADE:

INVERTED HAMSTRING

MUSCLES IT TARGETS:
HAMSTRINGS, GLUTES

HOW TO DO IT: Stand on your left leg, your knee bent slightly, and raise your right leg off the floor. Raise your arms out to the sides so that your body forms the letter "T", with your thumbs pointing up. Without changing the bend in your left knee, bend at your hips and lower your torso until it's parallel to the floor. As you bend over, make sure your arms remain out to your sides with your thumbs pointing up. Your right leg should stay in line with your body as you lower your torso. Pause, then raise your torso back to the starting position. Switch legs after 15 seconds.

STANDARD EXERCISE:
PUSHUP POSITION DUMBBELL ROW
THE UPGRADE:

DUMBBELL PUSHUP AND ROW

MUSCLES IT TARGETS:
ABS, BACK, BICEPS, SHOULDERS, CHEST

HOW TO DO IT: Place a pair of hex dumbbells at the spot where you position your hands for a pushup. Grasp the dumbbell handles and set yourself in pushup position. Lower your body to the floor, pause, then push yourself back up. Once you're back in the starting position, row the dumbbell in your right hand to the side of your chest by pulling it upward and bending your arm. Pause, then lower the dumbbell back

down, and repeat the same movement with your left arm.
That's one repetition.

BONUS TOTAL BODY EXERCISE: DUMBBELL PLANK ARM RAISE

HOW TO DO IT: Grab a pair of hex dumbbells and assume a pushup
position, with your arms straight. Keeping your core stiff, reach forward
with your right arm. Try to prevent your body from rotating. Hold for
a few seconds and lower back down. Repeat with your left arm. That's
one rep. (If this is too hard, you can perform the move without dumbbells.) To make it harder, perform a pushup in between arm raises.

STANDARD EXERCISE:
DUMBBELL FRONT SQUAT

THE UPGRADE:
DUMBBELL OVERHEAD SQUAT

MUSCLES IT TARGETS:
QUADS, HAMSTRINGS, GLUTES, SHOULDERS, ABS

HOW TO DO IT: Hold a pair of dumbbells straight over your shoulders,
with your arms completely straight. Set your feet slightly wider than
hip-width apart and brace your core. Lower your body until your
thighs are at least parallel to the floor. Your lower back should stay
naturally arched for the entire movement—don't allow the dumbbell to
fall forward as you squat. Pause, and then push back to the starting
position.

STANDARD EXERCISE:
DUMBBELL PUSH PRESS

THE UPGRADE:
JUMP SQUAT WITH OVERHEAD REACH

MUSCLES IT TARGETS:
QUADS, HAMSTRINGS, GLUTES, SHOULDERS, CALVES

HOW TO DO IT: Place your hands at your sides, push your hips back,
bend your knees, and lower your body until your upper thighs are
parallel to the floor. Pause, then jump as high as you can. As you
jump into the air, press your hands above your head as far as you can
so that your arms are fully extended. After landing, and then
immediately squat down again and repeat.

STANDARD EXERCISE:
DUMBBELL HANG PULL
THE UPGRADE:

DUMBBELL JUMP SHRUG

MUSCLES IT TARGETS:
QUADS, HAMSTRINGS, GLUTES, SHOULDERS, TRAPEZIUS, CALVES
HOW TO DO IT: Grab a pair of dumbbells and let them hang at arm's length, your palms facing your sides. Bend at your hips and knees until the dumbbells hang just below your knees. Simultaneously thrust your hips forward, shrug your shoulders forcefully, and jump as high as you can. Land as softly you can, reset, and repeat.

STANDARD EXERCISE:
CROSS-BODY MOUNTAIN CLIMBER
THE UPGRADE:

MOUNTAIN CLIMBER

MUSCLES IT TARGETS:
ABS, OBLIQUES
HOW TO DO IT: Assume a pushup position with your arms completely straight. Lift your right foot off the floor and slowly raise your knee as close to your chest as you can. Touch the floor with your right foot. Return to the starting position. Repeat with your left leg. Alternate back and forth for the selected time period.
BONUS ABS EXERCISE: Bird dog and rotate
HOW TO DO IT: Get down on all fours and place your right hand behind your head. Extend your left leg straight out behind you. Bring your right elbow and left knee underneath your body so that they touch. Extend them both back to the starting position, and look over your right shoulder. Repeat on the other side. Focus on maintaining a strong core and strong glutes so your entire body is stable.

STANDARD EXERCISE:
ALTERNATING SPLIT-JUMP
THE UPGRADE:

DUMBBELL LUNGE

MUSCLES IT TARGETS:
QUADS, GLUTES, HAMSTRINGS
HOW TO DO IT: Grab a pair of dumbbells and hold them at arm's length next to your sides, your palms facing each other. Step forward with your left leg and slowly lower your body until your front knee is bent at least 90 degrees. Pause, then push yourself to the starting position as quickly as you can. Repeat with your right leg.

STANDARD EXERCISE:
T-STABILIZER

THE UPGRADE:

ALTERNATING SIDE PLANK

MUSCLES IT TARGETS:
ABS, OBLIQUES

HOW TO DO IT: Lie on your left side with your knees straight. Prop your upper body up on your left forearm. Brace your core by contracting your abs forcefully, as if you were about to be punched in the belly. Raise your hips until your body forms a straight line from your ankles to your shoulders. This is a side plank. Hold for a moment and then rotate your body so you're resting all your weight on both of your elbows and your body forms a straight line from your shoulders to your ankles. Hold for another moment, and then rotate onto your right forearm and perform another side plank. Keep rotating through all three planks until time is up.

STANDARD EXERCISE:
DUMBBELL LUNGE AND ROTATION

THE UPGRADE:

DUMBBELL REVERSE LUNGE AND ROTATIONAL PRESS

MUSCLES IT TARGETS:
QUADS, GLUTES, HAMSTRINGS, OBLIQUES, SHOULDER

HOW TO DO IT: Grab a dumbbell with your left hand and hold it next to your left shoulder, your palm facing in. Step backward with your left leg and lower your body into a reverse lunge as you simultaneously press the dumbbell straight above your left shoulder. As you press the dumbbell overhead, rotate your torso to the right. Return to the starting position, shift the dumbbell in your right hand, and repeat on the other side.

STANDARD EXERCISE:
DUMBBELL ROW

THE UPGRADE:

ALTERNATING DUMBBELL ROW

MUSCLES IT TARGETS:
BACK, BICEPS

HOW TO DO IT: Grab a pair of dumbbells, bend at your hips and knees, and lower your torso until it's almost parallel to the floor. Let the dumbbells hang at arm's length from your shoulders, your palms facing behind you. Instead of rowing both dumbbells up at once, lift them one at a time in an alternating fashion. As you lift one dumbbell, lower the other without allowing your back to round.

100 Ways to Burn 100 Calories

What follows are some of the most creative and surprising ways that we could find to dispense with calories. Who knew fighting fat could be so much fun?

1. Slather on lip balm 765 times.
2. Relive the '80s: Lip-sync George Michael's "Faith" 16 times.
3. DVR an episode of *30 Rock* and watch it commercial-free. (Laughing for 10 minutes straight can burn 40 calories—no joke.)
4. Watch a documentary like *Food Inc.*, *The Cove*, or *An Inconvenient Truth*. (Serious stuff doesn't scorch as many calories.)
5. Wiggle while you watch TV for 40 minutes: Fidgeters burn up to 350 more calories a day than couch potatoes.
6. Get off your butt 33 times to change the channel.
7. Use the remote to channel surf for 68 minutes.
8. Surf for real for 34 minutes.
9. Fly a kite for 20 minutes.
10. Play beach volleyball for 13 minutes.
11. Bounce a volleyball on your knee 600 times.
12. Spend 17 minutes wrestling a beach ball away from your boyfriend.
13. Carry a cooler stocked with three bottles of water, a six-pack, four PB&Js, two oranges, a bag of tortilla chips, and 12 servings of salsa for 22 minutes.
14. Find the perfect teeny-weeny polka-dot bikini: Try on 16 suits (one every 3 minutes).
15. Polka for real for 23 minutes.
16. Do the horizontal polka missionary-style for 1 hour and 7 minutes.

17. Spice things up with 35 minutes of foreplay and 45 minutes of sex in different positions.
18. Ride him like a cowgirl for 26 minutes (straddling requires more calorie-burning leg work).
19. Swing a lasso over your head 375 times.
20. Milk a cow for 34 minutes.
21. Shear three sheep (6 minutes per sheep).
22. Fish for 41 minutes.
23. Make like a fish and swim at a leisurely pace for 17 minutes.
24. Do 250 breaststrokes (about 10 minutes).
25. Indulge your inner dork and do 27 underwater handstands.
26. Dog-paddle for 17 minutes.
27. Walk a toy poodle for 41 minutes (at 2 miles per hour).
28. Let a Great Dane walk you for 13 minutes (5 mph).
29. Learn to "walk the dog": Yo-yo for 25 minutes.
30. Alternate between cat pose, cow pose, and downward dog 13 times, holding each for 30 seconds.
31. Walk up 33 flights of stairs.
32. Strap on 4-inch stilettos and you only have to climb up 25 flights.
33. Hit the stair climber for 11 minutes.
34. Push a grocery cart for 45 minutes.
35. Put a 42-pound 4-year-old in the cart's child seat and push it for half an hour.
36. Opt for self-checkout: Wait in line for 7 minutes, ring yourself up for another 10, bag your own grub, and load up the car.
37. Carry five grocery bags from the car to the kitchen and put the food away, take out the trash, wash the dishes, and wipe down the kitchen counter.
38. Eat chili for a couple of days: Research shows that chili

peppers boost your metabolic rate, burning 50 more calories a day.

39. Chew calorie-free gum for 9 hours.

40. Wash, halve, and seed two acorn squash, then watch them bake for 30 minutes.

41. Play squash for 8 minutes.

42. Play "Chopsticks" on the piano incessantly for 41 minutes.

43. Eat four meals with chopsticks instead of a fork: Slowing down can help you consume about 25 fewer calories per meal.

44. Lift and lower a soy sauce bottle 170 times with your right hand and a wok 170 times with your left.

45. Take a leisurely walk in the park for 51 minutes.

46. Walk backward in the park for 43 minutes.

47. Walk with hiking poles for 22 minutes—you'll burn 20 percent more calories.

48. Pole-vault for 17 minutes.

49. Sing the *Grease* original soundtrack from start to finish.

50. Degrease by scrubbing in the shower for 15 minutes, then spend 7 minutes shaving, 3 minutes toweling off, 4 minutes moisturizing, and 20 minutes blow-drying and styling your hair.

51. Shop during your lunch hour while carrying a 7-pound hobo bag (and, naturally, a few new purchases).

52. Have fun when you get back to work: Twirl 123 times in your office chair (try not to puke).

53. E-mail for 68 minutes.

54. Get casual for 4 days: A study shows that people take 491 more steps and burn 25 more calories on days when they wear jeans to work.

55. Go backpacking for 15 minutes.

56. Strap a parachute to your back and spend 30 minutes skydiving over the volcanoes in Tongariro National Park, New Zealand.

57. Land in the Taupo Volcanic Zone and climb 26 percent of the way up in 18 minutes.

58. Cool down with 20 minutes of white-water rafting in the nearby Tongariro River.

59. Take in the greenery: Sit in lotus position and breathe deeply for 1 hour and 42 minutes.

60. Drink three cups of green tea in 24 hours: Researchers say it can increase energy expenditure by 106 calories.

61. Chug twelve 8-ounce glasses of ice water a day (it has the same effect on your metabolism as green tea).

62. Go 20 miles per hour on your bike for 6½ minutes.

63. Stay up on a unicycle for 20 minutes.

64. Ride a bike built for two for 12 minutes.

65. Ask your guy to massage you for 1 hour and 50 minutes.

66. Pay him back with a 25-minute rubdown.

67. Play Twister for 1 hour and 8 minutes.

68. Play Nintendo for 41 minutes.

69. Better yet, get moving with the GameCube's Dance Dance Revolution: Mario Mix for 24 minutes. (Turn on the workout feature to see how many calories you've burned.)

70. If you're more sports goddess than cha-cha dancer, play interactive Wii Tennis for 13 minutes.

71. No game necessary: Do 780 jumping jacks. Yes, 780.

72. Make like Laila Ali and jump rope as fast as you can for 8 minutes.

73. Jump on a trampoline for 29 minutes.

74. Jog on the treadmill at 4 mph for 25 minutes or at 7 mph for 9 minutes.

75. Run 5 percent of a marathon at a 10-minute-per-mile pace.

76. Wait in an airport security line for 15 minutes, walk through the metal detector once, lift and lower a 40-pound suitcase twice, then run for 3 minutes to catch your flight (stupid lines!).

77. Fill out 86 luggage tags.

78. Tag along with a mail carrier for 6 percent of her route. Mail carriers take about 18,904 steps a day, four times more than the average American.

79. Accompany a nurse on her rounds for half an hour—she logs about 8,648 steps.

80. Nurse your newborn for 30 minutes.

81. Nurse a hangover: Sleep in for 1 hour and 53 minutes.

82. Read Capote's *Breakfast at Tiffany's* from start to finish.

83. Kick off your Sunday shoes and dance to the first four songs off the *Footloose* soundtrack.

84. Spend 29 minutes mopping over any scuff marks.

85. Rearrange your furniture for 17 minutes.

86. Sweep your floors for 15 minutes, then vacuum for 15.

87. Dirt Devil your car mats for 5 minutes, then wax your ride for 20.

88. When you fill 'er up, walk into the station to pay, 23 times.

89. Cut your lawn with a push mower for 17 minutes.

90. Push a power mower instead for 23.

91. Brush your teeth for 2 minutes, 25 times.

92. Floss and gargle with Listerine after each brushing and you'll burn another 100.

93. Smile for the camera: Shoot pictures for 35 minutes.

94. Say cheesy! Hula-hoop for 22 minutes.

95. Crank your iPod as you walk at 3.5 mph for 23 minutes. (Studies show that listening to music makes you walk off more calories.)

96. Go retro: Roller-skate for 15 minutes.

97. Show off your bowling skills for 34 minutes.

98. Spend 53 minutes learning the French alphabet.

99. Now read 30 pages of Hugo's *Les Misérables*.

100. Read numbers 1 to 100 nine more times.

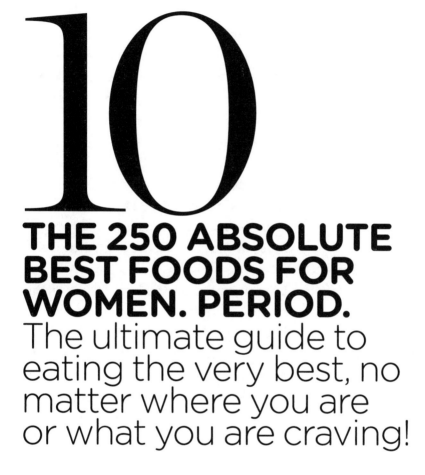

10

THE 250 ABSOLUTE BEST FOODS FOR WOMEN. PERIOD.
The ultimate guide to eating the very best, no matter where you are or what you are craving!

The best things in life generally aren't free. In fact, they'll likely set you back a few big ones. We're talking about the diamonds, the handbags, the Jimmy Choos.

But what if we told you that you are entitled to the best, no matter what? And that the best doesn't have to damage your bottom line—not the one in your bank account and not the one squeezing into those high-end jeans, either.

When it comes to having the absolute best—no compromises, no excuses—there's one way you can score big without breaking your calorie bank: You can—you will—eat the very best food in the world.

We know what you're thinking: a list of the best foods is going to contain nothing but piddling protein bars and tasteless tempeh patties. What could be more unappetizing?

But that's not the point of this list. This list is designed to be your go-to guide no matter what you're craving. Jonesing for some chips and salsa after work (and a bottle of beer to wash it down)? They're on there. No energy to make anything more than a frozen burrito for dinner? We've got you covered. Craving a little fro-yo before bedtime? Check.

In fact, you won't believe some of the things you'll find on this list: bacon cheese burgers, doughnuts, banana splits. We've even included the best items to order at restaurants—if you're heading to P.F. Chang's with some pals, check out the dumplings we've selected for you. As publishers of the *Eat This, Not That!* series of nutrition guides, we have access to the largest database of foods ever assembled. We've tested and tasted every single one of these items, and they all meet the high standards of the *Women's Health* Nutrition System. Eggroll? Margarita? Cheesesteak? If you simply have to have one, these are the ones you should have, and you'll still lose fat, build lean muscle, and sculpt the body you want. And while calories were a big part of our calculations, we refused to compromise on taste or on nutritional content—a few extra grams of protein and fiber are usually worth a few dozen calories.

So go ahead, aim high and treat yourself to the best food on the planet. Your body—and your tastebuds—will thank you.

THE VERY BEST FOODS AT THE SUPERMARKET

BREADS AND GRAINS

1. Best Cereal
Kashi Whole-Wheat Biscuits, Cinnamon Harvest
One bowl contains all the fiber you need to stay full until lunch.
PER 2 OZ (28 BISCUITS): 180 calories, 6 g protein, 43 g carbs (5 g fiber, 9 g sugars), 1 g fat, 0 g sodium

2. Best Instant Oatmeal
Quaker Weight Control Instant Oatmeal, Cinnamon
This morning meal has a sane number of calories and won't jolt your taste buds with too much sugar.
PER PACKET: 160 calories, 7 g protein, 29 g carbs (6 g fiber, 1 g sugars), 3 g fat, 290 mg sodium

3. Best Steel-Cut Oats
Arrowhead Mills Organic Steel Cut Oats Hot Cereal
It's nuttier and more filling than instant oatmeal.
PER ¼ CUP: 160 calories, 6 g protein, 27 g carbs (8 g fiber, 0 g sugars), 3 g fat, 0 mg sodium

4. Best Granola
Nature's Path Organic Pomegran Plus Granola with Cherries
Mix into Greek yogurt (# 31) for an easy postworkout snack.
PER ¾ CUP: 250 calories, 5 g protein, 38 g carbs (4 g fiber, 13 g sugars), 9 g fat, 60 mg sodium

5. Best Breakfast Bar
KIND Plus Almond Cashew + Flax (Omega-3)
A crunchy, craving-busting bar with just nine ingredients—all of which you can pronounce.
PER BAR: 150 calories, 4 g protein, 18 g carbs (4 g fiber, 14 g sugars), 9 g fat, 0 mg sodium

6. Best Bagel
Pepperidge Farm Whole Grain
Include a scrambled egg with one of these for a protein-packed start to your day.
PER BAGEL: 250 calories, 11 g protein, 49 g carbs (6 g fiber, 9 g sugars), 1.5 g fat, 450 mg sodium

7. Best English Muffin
Rudi's Organic Whole Grain Wheat English Muffins
Upgrade your breakfast: Top it with tomato, egg, and a slice of Swiss (#23).
PER MUFFIN: 120 calories, 5 g protein, 23 g carbs (3 g fiber, 2 g sugars), 1 g fat, 220 mg sodium

8. Best Sliced Bread
Arnold Grains & More Bread, 100% Whole Wheat Triple Health
No high-fructose corn syrup and plenty of fiber.
PER SLICE: 100 calories, 4 g protein, 20 g carbs (6 g fiber, 3 g sugars), 2 g fat, 170 mg sodium

217

9. Best Burger Bun
Arnold Select Sandwich Thins, Whole Wheat

Don't let the bread overwhelm your sandwich. These thin buns save on calories so you can layer on protein.

PER BUN: 100 calories, 5 g protein, 21 g carbs (5 g fiber, 2 g sugars), 1 g fat, 230 mg sodium

10. Best Hot Dog Roll
Pepperidge Farm Classic Whole Grain White

A tasty bun that stands up to whatever you top your dog with.

PER ROLL: 110 calories, 6 g protein, 21 g carbs (2 g fiber, 2 g sugars), 1 g fat, 220 mg sodium

11. Best Tortilla
La Tortilla Factory Smart & Delicious Extra Virgin Olive Oil Multi-Grain Soft Wrap

Wrap slices of avocado, lettuce, tomato, and cooked bacon (#115) in this tortilla for an awesome riff on a BLT.

PER TORTILLA: 100 calories, 9 g protein, 18 g carbs (12 g fiber, 1 g sugars), 3.5 g fat, 290 mg sodium

12. Best Pita
Weight Watchers 100% Whole Wheat

Perfect for a sandwich on the go.

PER PITA: 100 calories, 7 g protein, 24 g carbs (9 g fiber, 0 g sugars), 1 g fat, 260 mg sodium

13. Best Pizza Crust
Rustic Crust Organic Great Grains

Think outside the box: Top your pizza with thinly sliced potatoes, chopped leeks, prosciutto, and blue cheese crumbles. Bake at 450°F for 15 minutes or until crispy.

PER ⅛ CRUST: 140 calories, 5 g protein, 28 g carbs (5 g fiber, 0 g sugars), 1.5 g fat, 190 mg sodium

14. Best Whole-Wheat Pasta
Bionaturae Organic Whole Wheat Spaghetti

A whole-wheat pasta that doesn't taste like the box from which it came.

PER 2 OZ: 180 calories, 7 g protein, 35 g carbs (6 g fiber, 1 g sugars), 1.5 g fat, 0 mg sodium

15. Best Regular Pasta
Ronzoni Smart Taste Thin Spaghetti

It's smart because it has as much calcium as a glass of milk and three times the fiber of regular pasta.

PER 2 OZ: 180 calories, 6 g protein, 43 g carbs (7 g fiber, 1 g sugars), 0.5 g fat, 5 mg sodium

16. Best Quick-Cooking Rice
Uncle Ben's Ready Whole Grain Brown

The easiest side dish ever. Microwave for 90 seconds and you're good to go.

PER CUP: 240 calories, 5 g protein, 39 g carbs (2 g fiber, 0 g sugars), 3 g fat, 15 mg sodium

17. Best Grain

Bob's Red Mill Organic Whole Grain Quinoa

Switch up your sides by swapping it for rice.

PER ¼ CUP: 170 calories, 7 g protein, 30 g carbs (3 g fiber, 0 g sugars), 2.5 g fat, 2 mg sodium

18. Best Flour

King Arthur Flour 100% Organic Unbleached White Whole Wheat

Rich in fiber just like regular whole-wheat flour but with a lighter flavor. Perfect for making homemade pizza dough.

PER ¼ CUP: 100 calories, 4 g protein, 18 g carbs (3 g fiber, <1 g sugars), 0.5 g fat, 0 mg sodium

DAIRY AND DELI

19. Best Milk

Organic Valley Reduced Fat 2%

A little fat in your milk may help you absorb vitamins.

PER CUP: 130 calories, 8 g protein, 13 g carbs (0 g fiber, 12 g sugars), 5 g fat, 125 mg sodium

20. Best Chocolate Milk

Horizon Reduced Fat 2%

Drink this postworkout: Its combo of carbs and protein can help repair your muscles.

PER CUP: 180 calories, 8 g protein, 27 g carbs (<1 fiber, 27 g sugars), 5 g fat, 160 mg sodium

21. Best All-Purpose Cheese

Bella Rosa Parmigiano Reggiano

Grate this sharp Italian cheese on everything from pasta to pizza to soup.

PER GRATED TBSP: 20 calories, 2 g protein, N/A carbs, 1.5 g fat, N/A sodium

22. Best High-End Cheese

Emmi Le Gruyere Cave-Aged Kaltbach

Pair this rich and luscious cheese (available in many supermarkets) with an apple for the ultimate snack.

PER OZ: 120 calories, 8 g protein, 0 g carbs, 9 g fat, 160 mg sodium

23. Best Sandwich Cheese

Jarlsberg Lite Reduced Fat Swiss Cheese, Deli Fresh Slices

Well-rounded flavor without the high sodium content of processed American cheese.

PER SLICE: 50 calories, 7 g protein, 0 g carbs, 2.5 g fat, 100 mg sodium

24. Best Shredded Cheese

Organic Valley Reduced Fat Monterey Jack Cheese

It tastes great and melts well, unlike other low-fat cheeses.

PER ¼ CUP: 80 calories, 8 g protein, 1 g carbs (0 g fiber, 0 g sugars), 5 g fat, 180 mg sodium

25. Best Snacking Cheese

Laughing Cow Mini
Babybel, Light
*Keep a few in your work tote (in an
insulated container) to fight on-the-
job hunger.*
PER PIECE: 50 calories, 6 g protein,
0 g carbs, 3 g fat, 160 mg sodium

26. Best Cream Cheese

Philadelphia Whipped
Cream Cheese
*With a third fewer calories than regu-
lar Philadelphia cream cheese—and
all the flavor—you can schmear without fear.*
PER 2 TBSP: 60 calories, 1 g protein,
1 g carbs (0 g fiber, <1 g sugars),
6 g fat, 90 mg sodium

27. Best Cottage Cheese

Friendship Lowfat
Cottage Cheese
*Our tasters noted this brand has more
curds and less liquid than others, for a
more satisfying snack.*
PER ½ CUP: 90 calories, 16 g protein,
3 g carbs (0 g fiber, 3 g sugars),
1 g fat, 360 mg sodium

28. Best Sour Cream

Breakstone's All Natural
*Stir in the juice and zest of a lime and
some chopped scallions to make an
awesome taco topping.*
PER 2 TBSP: 60 calories, 1 g protein,
1 g carbs (0 g fiber, 1 g sugars),
5 g fat, 10 mg sodium

29. Best Butter

Keller's Whipped Butter, Salted
*Big butter flavor, with more air
(hence fewer calories) than your typical stick of butter.*
PER TBSP: 70 calories, 0 g protein,
0 g carbs, 7 g fat, 55 mg sodium

30. Best Butter Spread

Keller's Spreadable Butter
with Canola Oil
*Our tasters agree: This brand
tastes like the real deal, and spreads
easily.*
PER TBSP: 100 calories, 0 g protein,
0 g carbs, 11 g fat, 80 mg sodium

31. Best Plain Yogurt

Stonyfield Farm Oikos
Organic Greek Yogurt, Plain
*Throw in some blueberries, and add a
drizzle of honey if you like your
yogurt sweet.*
PER 5.3-OZ CONTAINER: 80 calories,
15 g protein, 6 g carbs (0 g fiber,
6 g sugars), 0 g fat, 60 mg sodium

32. Best Flavored Yogurt

Chobani Nonfat Strawberry
Greek Yogurt
*Thick, creamy, and sweet. Think
of it as a healthy dessert.*
PER 6-OZ CONTAINER: 140 calories,
14 g protein, 20 g carbs (1 g fiber,
19 g sugars), 0 g fat, 65 mg sodium

33. Best Probiotic Yogurt

Lifeway Lowfat Raspberry Kefir
*This fruity, drinkable probiotic didn't
have a gross aftertaste like some of
the others we tried.*
PER CUP: 160 calories, 11 g protein,
25 g carbs (3 g fiber, 21 g sugars),
125 mg sodium

34. Best Eggs

Eggland's Best Organic

Fry one up for your morning toast: The rich yellow yolk packs great flavor.

PER LARGE EGG: 70 calories, 6 g protein, 0 g carbs, 4 g fat, 60 mg sodium

35. Best Cold Cuts

Applegate Farms Organic Roasted Turkey Breast

Juicy, flavorful deli turkey.

PER 2 OZ: 50 calories, 10 g protein, 1 g carbs (0 g fiber, 0 g sugars), 360 mg sodium

36. Best Pepperoni

Hormel Turkey 70% Less Fat

Perfect as an out-of-the-bag snack. More satisfying than potato chips, too.

PER 17 SLICES: 70 calories, 9 g protein, 0 g carbs, 4 g fat, 640 mg sodium

FROZEN FOODS

37. Best Frozen Appetizer

Annie Chun's Chicken & Garlic Mini Wontons

They're easier on your belly than mozzarella sticks.

PER 4 WONTONS: 60 calories, 3 g protein, 9 g carbs (1 g fiber, 1 g sugars), 0.5 g fat, 150 mg sodium

38. Best Beef Entrée

Stouffer's Beef Pot Roast

One of the few selections that tastes like beef. A little high on sodium, so watch your portions.

PER PACKAGE: 320 calories, 20 g protein, 41 g carbs (8 g fiber, 9 g sugars), 8 g fat, 1,570 mg sodium

39. Best Chicken Entrée

Kashi Red Curry Chicken

Miraculously, this Thai-inspired dish doesn't taste like a frozen meal, and the combo of sweet potato, bok choy, and kale adds flavor as well as fiber.

PER PACKAGE: 300 calories, 18 g protein, 40 g carbs (5 g fiber, 10 g sugars), 9 g fat, 470 mg sodium

40. Best Fish Entrée

Seapak Roasted Garlic Encrusted Flounder

For a great fish sandwich, pair with mayo (#74), lemon, and cilantro

PER FILLET: 300 calories, 19 g protein, 40 g carbs (1 g fiber, 14 g sugars), 7 g fat, 1,010 mg sodium

41. Best Pasta Entrée

Kashi Pesto Pasta Primavera

A good mix of whole-grain pasta, basil pesto, and an assortment of vegetables.

PER MEAL: 290 calories, 11 g protein, 37 g carbs (7 g fiber, 4 g sugars), 11 g fat, 750 mg sodium

42. Best Vegetarian Entrée

Amy's Black Bean Enchilada Dinner

Meatless protein from beans, corn, rice, and tofu combine for a satisfying Mexican meal that's way healthier than the typical burrito.

PER PACKAGE: 330 calories, 9 g protein, 53 g carbs (9 g fiber, 4 g sugars), 8 g fat, 740 mg sodium

43. Best Pizza
Amy's Cheese Pizza
Make it even tastier by adding thinly sliced onions and peppers two minutes before it's done.
PER ⅓ PIZZA: 290 calories, 12 g protein, 33 g carbs (2 g fiber, 4 g sugars), 12 g fat, 590 mg sodium

44. Best Burrito
Evol Burritos Cilantro Lime Chicken
Free-range chicken, organic black beans, real salsa. What's not to love?
PER BURRITO: 320 calories, 16 g protein, 49 g carbs (4 g fiber, 1 g sugars), 7 g fat, 450 mg sodium

45. Best Vegetarian Burger
Gardenburger GardenVegan
It's best cooked on the grill or in a skillet with a teaspoon of canola oil (#118). Top it with a few slices of fresh avocado.
PER PATTY: 80 calories, 9 g protein, 12 g carbs (4 g fiber, 0 g sugars), 1 g fat, 270 mg sodium

46. Best Fish Sticks
Dr. Praeger's Sensible Foods Fish Sticks, Potato Crusted
Try them sprinkled with lemon juice, freshly ground black pepper (#122), and chopped parsley for a more sophisticated meal.
PER 3 STICKS: 120 calories, 6 g protein, 7 g carbs (<1 g fiber, 0 g sugars), 8 g fat, 220 mg sodium

47. Best French Fries
Cascadian Farm Crinkle Cut French Fries
No partially hydrogenated oil (a.k.a. trans fat).
PER 18 PIECES: 110 calories, 2 g protein, 17 g carbs (2 g fiber, 1 g sugars), 4 g fat, 10 mg sodium

48. Best Breakfast Sandwich
Weight Watchers Smart Ones Morning Express Breakfast Quesadilla
A good source of protein and fiber—which means it'll keep you full until lunch.
PER QUESADILLA: 230 calories, 12 g protein, 29 g carbs (6 g fiber, 1 g sugars), 7 g fat, 730 mg sodium

49. Best Waffle
Van's 8 Whole Grains Multigrain
Top these fiber-rich waffles with yogurt (#31) and fruit for a satisfying breakfast.
PER 2 WAFFLES: 180 calories, 3 g protein, 31 g carbs (6 g fiber, 3 g sugars), 7 g fat, 320 mg sodium

50. Best Vegetable
Cascadian Farm Organic Garden Peas
You don't even need butter—these peas require only a pinch of sea salt (#121) to taste amazing.
PER ⅔ CUP: 70 calories, 4 g protein, 12 g carbs (4 g fiber, 4 g sugars), 0 g fat, 95 mg sodium

51. Best Fruit

Whole Foods 365 Everyday Value Organic Berry Blend
Keep a bag on hand for smoothies.
PER ¾ CUP: 70 calories, 1 g protein, 15 g carbs (3 g fiber, 10 g sugars), 0 g fat, 0 mg sodium

52. Best Ice Cream

Breyers Smooth & Dreamy All Natural ½ Fat Vanilla Bean
Skip the chunks and swirls. This ice cream has enough flavor to stand on its own.
PER ½ CUP: 110 calories, 3 g protein, 16 g carbs (0 g fiber, 16 g sugars), 3.5 g fat, 50 mg sodium

53. Best Frozen Treat

Edy's Fruit Bars (Variety Pack: Lime, Strawberry, Wildberry)
Real fruit trumps artificial flavor in a low-calorie pop. A great guilt-free snack.
PER BAR: 60 calories, 0 g protein, 13 g carbs (0 g fiber, 13 g sugars), 0 g fat, 0 mg sodium

JARRED AND CANNED GOODS

54. Best Soup

Lucini Italia Rustic Italian Minestrone Soup
Filled with chunks of hearty vegetables.
PER CUP: 160 calories, 5 g protein, 22 g carbs (4 g fiber, 6 g sugars), 7 g fat, 760 mg sodium

55. Best Chili

Amy's Organic Low-Fat Medium Black Bean
Plenty of fiber, with just the right amount of spice.
PER CUP: 200 calories, 13 g protein, 31 g carbs (13 g fiber, 3 g sugars), 3 g fat, 680 mg sodium

56. Best Refried Beans

Eden Organic Spicy Refried Black Beans
These spicy beans have more flavor than regular canned beans and, despite the "refried" part, only a bit of added fat.
PER ½ CUP: 110 calories, 6 g protein, 18 g carbs (7 g fiber, 0 g sugars), 1.5 g fat, 180 mg sodium

57. Best Canned Beans

Eden Organic Black Beans
Simmer these antioxidant-rich beans with sautéed onions and peppers for an easy side.
PER ½ CUP: 110 calories, 7 g protein, 18 g carbs (6 g fiber, 0 g sugars), 1 g fat, 15 mg sodium

58. Best Canned Tomatoes

Cento San Marzano Organic Peeled Tomatoes
Chop these tomatoes until slightly chunky for the perfect pizza sauce.
PER ½ CUP: 25 calories, 1 g protein, 5 g carbs (2 g fiber, 4 g sugars), 0 g fat, 20 mg sodium

59. Best Olives
Mezzetta Jalapeño
Stuffed Olives

Just one, straight out of the jar, makes an instant salty-spicy snack–or a great addition to a martini. For an amazing salsa, chop some up and mix them with diced tomatoes and cilantro.

PER OLIVE: 10 calories, N/A protein, 1 g carbs (N/A fibers, N/A sugars), 1 g fat, N/A sodium

60. Best Pickle
Woodstock Farms Organic
Kosher Whole Dill Pickles

Crispier and tastier than typical jarred varieties. Slide one of these alongside your next sandwich.

PER PICKLE: 10 calories, 0 g protein, 2 g carbs (0 g fiber, 0 g sugars), 0 g fat, 580 mg sodium

61. Best Ready-to-Eat Tuna
Starkist Tuna, Chunk Light
in Water

A perfect match for a toasted English muffin (#7).

PER 2.6-OZ POUCH: 80 calories, 18 g protein, 1 g carbs (1 g fiber, 0 g sugars), 0.5 g fat, 300 mg sodium

62. Best Ready-to-Eat Salmon
Bumble Bee Premium
Wild Pink Salmon

A good source of heart-healthy omega-3 fatty acids.

PER 2 OZ: 60 calories, 14 g protein, 0 g carbs, 1.5 g fat, 180 mg sodium

SPREADS, DIPS, AND TOPPINGS

63. Best Ketchup
Heinz Organic

This version of the classic ketchup tastes fresher and brighter than the nonorganic variety.

PER TBSP: 20 calories, 5 g carbs (0 g fiber, 4 g sugars), 0 g fat, 190 mg sodium

64. Best Mustard
Annie's Naturals Organic
Dijon Mustard

Spread it on a sandwich instead of mayo, or make a quick homemade salad dressing: Blend ½ tablespoon of mustard and two tablespoons of lemon juice, then whisk in ¼ cup extra-virgin olive oil (#119) until smooth. Season with salt and freshly ground pepper.

PER TBSP: 5 calories, 0 g protein, 1 g carbs (N/A fiber, N/A sugars), 0 g fat, 120 mg sodium

65. Best Mayonnaise
Kraft with Olive Oil
Reduced Fat

For a killer spicy mayo that'll wake up your sandwich, combine this with hot sauce (#117) to taste.

PER TBSP: 45 calories, 2 g carbs (0 g fiber, 1 g sugars), 4 g fat, 95 mg sodium

66. **Best Barbecue Sauce**
Pork Barrel
Brush this relatively low-calorie sauce on chicken just minutes before it comes off the grill for a tangy, smoky flavor, or drizzle it over a roast-pork sandwich.
PER 2 TBSP: 35 calories, <1 g protein, 8 g carbs (0 g fiber, 7 g sugars), 390 mg sodium

67. **Best Steak Sauce**
Peter Luger Steak House Old Fashioned Sauce
Upgrade your steak with the tangy, lightly spicy sauce from Brooklyn's iconic chophouse.
PER TBSP: 30 calories, 0 g protein, 7 g carbs (0 g fiber, 7 g sugars), 0 g fat, 125 mg sodium

68. **Best Marinade**
Wild Thymes Tropical Mango Lime
It gives fish, chicken, other meats, and vegetables a flavor kick without adding too many calories.
PER TBSP: 12 calories, <1 g protein, 3 g carbs (1 g fiber, 2 g sugars), 0 g fat, 31 mg sodium

69. **Best Tomato Sauce**
La Famiglia DelGrosso Pasta Sauce, Chef John's Tomato Basil Masterpiece
It tastes like fresh tomatoes; not sugary like most jarred sauces.
PER ½ CUP: 70 calories, 1 g protein, 8 g carbs (2 g fiber, 5 g sugars), 4 g fat, 300 mg sodium

70. **Best Salsa**
Santa Barbara Salsa (Medium)
Unlike many other jarred and fresh salsas we tested, this one was not too sweet or salty, with a fresh, chunky texture.
PER OZ: 10 calories, 0 g protein, 2 g carbs (0 g fiber, 1 g sugars), 0 g fat, 170 mg sodium

71. **Best Guacamole**
Yucatan Organic Guacamole
Some "guacamole flavor" dips contain little actual avocado. This brand lists organic Hass avocados as the first ingredient.
PER 2 TBSP: 60 calories, 1 g protein, 3 g carbs (2 g fiber, 1 g sugars), 4.5 g fat, 170 mg sodium

72. **Best Peanut Butter**
Once Again Organic American Classic Creamy
Slather on a waffle (#49) for a tasty and filling breakfast.
PER 2 TBSP: 190 calories, 7 g protein, 7 g carbs (2 g fiber, 2 g sugars), 15 g fat, 55 mg sodium

73. **Best Jam/Fruit Spread**
Dickinson's Organic Strawberry Fruit Spread
Spoon onto vanilla ice cream (#52) for the perfect sundae.
PER TBSP: 45 calories, 0 g protein, 11 g carbs (0 g fiber, 11 g sugars), 0 g fat, 0 mg sodium

74. Best Condiment
Flora Sundried Tomato Bruschetta

Brush on baguette slices and top with fresh mozzarella, prosciutto, and basil, or stir into pasta with roasted vegetables.

PER 2 TBSP: 150 calories, 7 g protein, <1 g carbs (0 g fiber, <1 g sugars), 13 g fat, 190 mg sodium

75. Best Dip
Summer Fresh Baba Ghanouj Creamy Roasted Eggplant Dip

This smooth Middle Eastern dip tastes great with warmed pita.

PER 2 TBSP: 110 calories, 1 g protein, 1 g carbs (0 g fiber, 0 g sugars), 12 g fat, 180 mg sodium

76. Best Hummus
Cedar's Original Hommus Tahini

Creamy, with a punch of garlic. Add a drizzle of olive oil (#119) to enhance the flavors.

PER 2 TBSP: 60 calories, 2 g protein, 4 g carbs (1 g fiber, 1 g sugars), 4.5 g fat, 115 mg sodium

77. Best Salad Dressing
Drew's Roasted Garlic & Peppercorn Salad Dressing

Unlike most creamy dressings, this one's light enough not to clobber the flavor of the rest of the salad.

PER TBSP: 70 calories, 0 g protein, 0 g carbs, 8 g fat, 69 mg sodium

78. Best Pancake Syrup
Spring Tree 100% Pure All Natural Maple Syrup Grade A Dark Amber

Real maple syrup doesn't have high-fructose corn syrup or a cloying aftertaste.

PER TBSP: 53 calories, 13 carbs

SNACKS

79. Best Pretzel
Herr's Pretzel Sticks, Whole Grain, Honey Wheat

The fiber in this snack will help fill you up.

PER 7 PRETZELS: 110 calories, 3 g protein, 22 g carbs (4 g fiber, 2 g sugars), 1 g fat, 300 mg sodium

80. Best Tortilla Chip
Miguel's Organic Everything Tortilla Dippers

Our tasters went back for seconds.

PER 10 CHIPS: 140 calories, 2 g protein, 18 g carbs (2 g fiber, 0 g sugars), 7 g fat, 80 mg sodium

81. Best Potato Chip
Pop Chips Cheddar Potato

Popped with air, not fried, for a better sandwich side.

PER 20 CHIPS: 120 calories, 2 g protein, 20 g carbs (1 g fiber, 1 g sugars), 4 g fat, 290 mg sodium

82. Best Cracker
Kashi Original 7 Grain Snack Crackers

Dip into hummus (#76) for a healthy mid-afternoon snack.

PER 15 CRACKERS: 120 calories, 3 g protein, 21 g carbs (2 g fiber, 3 g sugars), 3.5 g fat, 160 mg sodium

83. **Best Popcorn**
Half Naked Popcorn
(made with olive oil)
Air-popped and dressed with just a touch of heart-healthy olive oil, it's the perfect movie snack.
PER 4 CUPS: 120 calories, 3 g protein, 21 g carbs (4 g fiber, 4 g sugars), 3 g fat, 140 mg sodium

84. **Best Jerky**
Matador Beef Jerky, Original
Pack it in your gym bag—jerky is a delicious on-the-go fat-fighting protein snack.
PER OZ: 80 calories, 11 g protein, 6 g carbs (0 g fiber, 5 g sugars), 1.5 g fat, 610 mg sodium

85. **Best Nut**
Planters Nut-rition Almonds
For an instant tummy-filling snack, reach for these nuts, seasoned only with sea salt.
PER 28 G (ABOUT 2 TBSP):
170 calories, 6 g protein, 6 g carbs (3 g fiber, 1 g sugars), 15 g fat, 40 mg sodium

86. **Best Nut Alternative**
Eden Organic Pumpkin Seeds
A high-protein snack you can take anywhere.
PER ¼ CUP: 200 calories, 10 g protein, 5 g carbs (5 g fiber, 0 g sugars), 16 g fat, 100 mg sodium

87. **Best Dried Fruit**
Peeled Snacks
Much-Ado-About-Mango
No added sugar or artificial flavors, and only one ingredient: mango.
PER 1.4-OZ BAG: 120 calories, 2 g protein, 28 g carbs (2 g fiber, 20 g sugars), 0 g fat, 0 mg sodium

88. **Best Trail Mix**
Sahale Snacks
Southwest Cashews
Not your forest ranger's gorp: This tangy mix is flavored with chili powder and cheddar cheese.
PER ¼ CUP: 140 calories, 5 g protein, 10 g carbs (1 g fiber, 3 g sugars), 10 g fat, 270 mg sodium

89. **Best Snack Bar**
Lärabar Peanut Butter Cookie
The perfect way to power through to a late lunch.
PER BAR: 220 calories, 7 g protein, 23 g carbs (4 g fiber, 18 g sugars), 12 g fat, 45 mg sodium

90. **Best Chocolate Bar**
Dagoba's Organic
Beacoup Berries
Dried fruit boosts flavor and antioxidants.
PER BAR: 250 calories, 5 g protein, 27 g carbs (7 g fiber, 18 g sugars), 19 g fat, 0 mg sodium

91. **Best Cookie**
Country Choice Organic
Soft Baked Double Fudge
Brownie Cookies
Rich and chewy—without calorie overload.
PER COOKIE: 90 calories, 1 g protein, 16 g carbs (1 g fiber, 10 g sugars), 3 g fat, 80 mg sodium

DRINKS

92. Best Bottled Water

Fiji

When you're not pouring purified water into a reusable canteen, pick up this water: Our tasters preferred its clean, crisp flavor above other brands.

0 calories

93. Best Sports Drink

Zico Pure Coconut Water with Mango

An 11-ounce serving packs more potassium than a banana (and a lot more than your average sports drink), all for a modest calorie count.

PER 11 OZ: 60 calories, 1 g protein, 15 g carbs (0 g fiber, 14 g sugars), 0 g fat, 60 mg sodium

94. Best Flavored Water

Poland Spring Sparkling Water with Lemon Essence

Kick your soda cravings for good with this carbonated water that has a hint of flavoring but no sugar.

0 calories

95. Best Fruit Juice

Simply Grapefruit

Naturally lower in sugar than other fruit juices and loaded with lycopene, it's the most underrated juice in the cooler. Mix it with sparkling water (#94) for a healthy riff on soda.

PER 8 OZ: 90 calories, 1 g protein, 21 g carbs (0 g fiber, 18 g sugars), 0 g fat, 10 mg sodium

96. Best Vegetable Juice

V8 100% Vegetable Juice, Low Sodium

This low-salt version (only 140 milligrams of sodium per cup) actually tastes better than the full-sodium version.

PER 8 OZ: 50 calories, 2 g protein, 10 carbs (2 g fiber, 8 g sugars), 0 g fat, 140 mg sodium

97. Best Bottled Smoothie

Bolthouse Farms Berry Boost

Not eating enough fruit? Drink this blend of blackberries, boysenberries, and raspberries.

PER 8 OZ: 130 calories, 0 g protein, 30 g carbs (4 g fiber, 21 g sugars), 1 g fat, 20 mg sodium

98. Best Bottled Tea

Honest Tea Organic Honey Green Tea

This tea has more metabolism-boosting, cancer-fighting catechins than its competitors.

PER 8 OZ: 35 calories, 0 g protein, 9 g carbs (0 g fiber, 9 g sugars), 5 mg sodium

99. Best Caffeinated Bag Tea

Numi Organic Aged Earl Grey Black Tea

This aged tea is more robust than your grandma's variety and bold enough to sub in for your morning coffee.

0 calories

100. Best Herbal Bag Tea

Stash Peppermint

Peppermint packs disease-fighting antioxidants and may help calm an upset stomach.

0 calories

101. Best Coffee
Illy Ground Coffee
A dark roast that brews up beautifully.
0 calories

102. Best Instant Coffee
Starbucks VIA Ready Brew
Be your own barista: Pour a packet into your mug, add hot water, and stir. No pot needed.
0 calories

103. Best Beer
Hoegaarden
A light-bodied Belgian brew with hints of spice and orange. It'll satisfy beer snobs—and regular folks, too.
PER 11.2 OZ: 176 calories, N/A protein, 13.4 g carbs (N/A fiber, N/A sugars), N/A fat, N/A sodium

104. Best Microbrew
Bell's Hopslam
This microbrewery's intense double India pale ale is flavorful and satisfyingly bitter. It deserves to be savored.
PER 12 OZ: 280 calories, N/A protein, N/A carbs (N/A fiber, N/A sugars), N/A fat, N/A sodium

105. Best Low-Calorie Beer
Guinness Draught
Dark does not equal heavy. This smooth Irish brew may have a few more calories than most light beers, but it also packs much more satisfaction.
PER 12 OZ: 126 calories, N/A protein, 10 g carbs (N/A fiber, N/A sugars), N/A fat, N/A sodium

106. Best Red Wine Under $20
Louis M. Martini Cabernet Sauvignon, Sonoma County, 2007
Delivers rich flavors of black cherry, blackberry, and fresh sage—and won't make a big dent in your paycheck.
PER 4 OZ: 98 calories, N/A protein, 4 g carbs, (N/A fiber, N/A sugars), N/A fat, N/A sodium

107. Best White Wine Under $15
Pacific Rim Dry Riesling, Columbia Valley, 2007
This versatile bargain bottle grabbed our attention with the apricot flavors that stand up even to Thai takeout.
PER 4 OZ: 86 calories, 1 g carbs

PROTEIN

108. Best Hot Dog
Applegate Farms Uncured Beef Hot Dogs
No nitrates means less chance that you'll develop a postmeal headache.
PER DOG: 80 calories, 5 g protein, 0 g carbs, 6 g fat, 380 mg sodium

109. Best Chicken
Bell & Evans Organic Boneless/Skinless Breast Meat
The juiciest, most flavorful supermarket poultry we tasted.
PER 4 OZ: 120 calories, 27 g protein, 0 g carbs, 1.5 g fat, 70 mg sodium

110. Best Steak

Laura's Lean Beef
Ribeye Steak
Lean and succulent.

PER 4 OZ: 175 calories, 24 g protein, 0 g carbs, 9 g fat, 70 mg sodium

111. Best Ground Beef

Laura's Beef 92% Lean Ground
For great burgers, all this humanely raised meat needs is a dash of salt and pepper.

PER 4 OZ: 160 calories, 21 g protein, 0 g carbs, 9 g fat, 70 mg sodium

112. Best Turkey

Diestel Boneless, Skinless
Turkey, Dark Meat
Diestel's turkeys are plumped on a natural vegetarian diet.

PER 4 OZ: 130 calories, 23 g protein, 0 g carbs, 3 g fat, 80 mg sodium

113. Best Specialty Meat

Great Range Ground Bison
Make this lean, robust meat your new secret ingredient in Super Bowl party chili.

PER 4 OZ: 190 calories, 20 g protein, 0 g carbs, 11 g fat, 60 mg sodium

114. Best Bacon

Oscar Mayer Center Cut
Naturally Smoked
Don't fear bacon—it's low in calories. You need only a couple of strips to add flavor to potato salad, pizza, or soup.

PER 3 SLICES: 70 calories, 7 g protein, 0 g carbs, 4.5 g fat, 270 mg sodium

115. Best Sausage

Al Fresco Sundried Tomato
Chicken Sausage with Basil
and Tomatoes
Split a link in half and broil it until the top begins to caramelize. Sprinkle with chopped cilantro and lime juice. Enjoy.

PER LINK: 140 calories, 15 g protein, 2 g carbs (0 g fiber, 2 g sugars), 7 g fat, 480 mg sodium

116. Best Protein Powder

At Large Nutrition
Nitrean Vanilla
A whey-casein blend that tastes good going down.

PER 30 G SCOOP: 113 calories, 23 g protein, 3 g carbs (N/A g fiber, N/A g sugars), 1 g fat, 95 mg sodium

COOKING STAPLES

117. Best Hot Sauce

Huy Fong Foods Tuong Ot
Sriracha
Made from hot chilies, this sauce delivers a burn that enhances every-thing from scrambled eggs to chicken to salsa.

PER TBSP: 5 calories, 0 g protein, 1 g carbs (0 g fiber, 1 g sugars), 0 g fat, 100 mg sodium

118. Best Everyday Oil

Spectrum Organic Canola Oil
Its neutral taste is suitable for everyday cooking, and it has a well-balanced fatty acids profile, to help fight disease.

PER TBSP: 120 calories, 0 g protein, 0 g carbs, 14 g fat, 0 g sodium

119. Best High-End Olive Oil
Yellingbo Gold Extra
Virgin Olive Oil
This peppery, light-bodied oil tastes amazing drizzled on top of fresh pasta, mozzarella, or crusty bread.
PER TBSP: 120 calories, 0 g protein, 0 g carbs, 14 g fat, 0 mg sodium

120. Best Vinegar
Colavita Balsamic Vinegar
Mix ¼ cup of this with ½ cup of olive oil, chopped herbs, some shavings of Parmesan cheese (#21), salt, and pepper. Stir well for an easy vinaigrette.
PER TBSP: 15 calories, 0 g protein, 3 g carbs (0 g fiber, 3 g sugars), 0 g fat, 0 mg sodium

121. Best Salt
Maldon Sea Salt Flakes
This salt is perfect for heightening the flavors of fish, meat, or vegetables after they're cooked. Try it on a rib eye steak (#110) and taste the difference.
0 calories

122. Best Pepper
Simply Organic Whole
Black Peppercorns
Forget the pre-ground stuff in the shaker. Freshly ground pepper, combined with sea salt (#121), is the cornerstone of flavorful cooking. Use each to your taste.
0 calories

123. Best Bread Crumbs
Wel-Pac Japanese Style
Panko Bread Crumbs
A lighter, crunchier Japanese variety that's great sprinkled over sautéed string beans.
PER 28 G: 110 calories, 4 g protein, 20 carbs (1 g fiber, 1 g sugars), 1 g fat, 85 mg sodium

124. Best Low-Sodium Broth
Pacific Natural Foods
Organic Free-Range Chicken
Tastes like homemade, with far less sodium than most brands. Use it as a base for soups.
PER CUP: 15 calories, 2 g protein, 1 g carbs (0 g fiber, 0 g sugars), 0 g fat, 70 mg sodium

125. Best Soy Sauce
Kikkoman Less Sodium
Soy Sauce
Use it as a salt substitute in soups, marinades, and dressings to add a savory flavor to your meals .
PER TBSP: 10 calories, 1 g protein, 1 g carbs (0 g fiber, 0 g sugars), 0 g fat, 575 mg sodium

THE VERY BEST RESTAURANT FOODS

Cooking at home is almost always the best choice when it comes to keeping off the pounds. A University of Massachusetts study found that eating breakfast out instead of at home more than doubles your odds of obesity. Restaurant meals often bigger than home-cooked ones, and you're also vulnerable to an impulse buy at a drive-thru or convenience store. Still, ya gotta get out once in a while. When you do, try these...

BREAKFAST

1. Best Oatmeal
Au Bon Pain Apple-Cinnamon Oatmeal (medium, 12 oz)
Between the rolled oats and apples, this bowl packs nearly a quarter of your day's recommended fiber without being overly sweet.
280 calories, 8 g protein, 56 g carbs (7 g fiber, 14 g sugars), 4 g fat, 10 mg sodium

2. Best Breakfast Platter
Bob Evans Classic Breakfast (two eggs, two bacon strips, and one slice of French toast)
The unfortunate truth about breakfast platters is that they're typically big enough to feed a small army. This one achieves the same combo effect without the belly-busting calorie load.
498 calories, 20 g protein, 20 g carbs (1 g fiber, 11 g sugars), 33 g fat, 849 mg sodium

3. Best Breakfast Burrito
Carl's Jr. Bacon & Egg Burrito
Lighter breakfast burritos are out there, but if you want something sizeable enough to fill you up and substantial enough to pack a load of protein, this is the burrito for you.
550 calories, 29 g protein, 37 g carbs (1 g fiber, 1 g sugars), 31 g fat, 970 mg sodium

4. Best Pancake Breakfast
Denny's Hearty Wheat Pancakes (stack of two)
Denny's fortifies its batter with wheat bran to make a fiber-rich stack of flapjacks that will to quell your hunger better than buttermilk pancakes ever could.
310 calories, 10 g protein, 64 g carbs (8 g fiber, 2 g sugars), 1.5 g fat, 950 mg sodium

5. Best Waffle Breakfast
Bob Evans Belgian Waffle with Strawberry Topping
The lightest waffle you'll find at any fast-casual restaurant, and by choosing the strawberry topping over standard pancake syrup, you save almost 150 calories.
435 calories, 10 g protein, 75 carbs (4 g fiber, 29 g sugars), 10 g fat, 795 mg sodium

6. Best Doughnut
Dunkin' Donuts Sugar-Raised Donut
If you're craving an occasional doughnut, this one's your best bet—you won't find another with fewer than 200 calories.
230 calories, 3 g protein, 22 g carbs (1 g fiber, 4 g sugars), 14 g fat, 330 mg sodium

7. Best Filled Donut
Tim Hortons Strawberry-Filled Donut
The same strawberry-filled doughnut at Krispy Kreme carries twice the fat.
230 calories, 4 g protein, 36 g carbs (1 g fiber, 12 g sugars), 8 g fat, 220 mg sodium

8. Best Breakfast Pastry
Starbucks 8-Grain Roll
Starbucks might call this muffin-shaped breakfast bread a roll, but don't get confused: The protein and fiber counts make it a great way to start your morning.
350 calories, 10 g protein, 67 g carbs (5 g fiber, 17 g sugars), 8 g fat, 520 mg sodium

9. Best Cinnamon Roll
Krispy Kreme Cinnamon Bun
This cinnamon roll has a surprisingly low calorie count, especially compared with the Panera Bread version that clocks in with a walloping 620 calories.
260 calories, 3 g protein, 28 g carbs (< 1 fiber, 13 g sugars), 16 g fat, 125 mg sodium

10. Best Muffin
Starbucks Apple Bran Muffin
How do you pack 7 grams of fiber into a muffin? By including unrefined ingredients like whole-wheat flour and oats, along with apples, cherries, and cranberries.
350 calories, 6 g protein, 64 g carbs (7 g fiber, 34 g sugars), 9 g fat, 520 mg sodium

11. Best Croissant
Tim Hortons Plain Croissant
Croissants are always going to be high in saturated fat, so stick to the simplest variety and add a slice of ham for an extra hit of protein.
270 calories, 4 g protein, 23 g carbs (1 g fiber, 2 g sugars), 18 g fat, 210 mg sodium

12. Best Parfait
Bob Evans Blueberry-Banana Mini Fruit & Yogurt Parfait (6.7 oz)
Bob uses low-fat yogurt to minimize calories, and the bananas and blueberries on top deliver a healthy dose of fiber and antioxidants.
177 calories, 4 g protein, 39 g carbs (3 g fiber, 34 g sugars), 1 g fat, 61 mg sodium

13. Best Breakfast Sandwich
Subway Black Forest Ham, Egg, and Cheese Muffin Melt
Big hits of protein and fiber—not to mention an astonishingly low calorie count—make this the one of the best breakfast creations out there. Plus Subway offers something no other fast-food joint does: unlimited vegetables on your sandwich.
180 calories, 15 g protein, 18 g carbs (5 g fiber, 1 g sugars), 7 g fat, 650 mg sodium

14. Best Breakfast Flatbread
Dunkin' Donuts Egg White and Turkey-Sausage Flatbread
This sandwich boasts two sources of lean protein, egg whites and turkey sausage, so it's sure to fuel you all morning long.
290 calories, 21 g protein, 34 carbs (3 g fiber, 6 g sugars), 8 g fat, 600 mg sodium

15. Best Whole-Egg Omelet
Denny's Veggie-Cheese Omelette
An industry-wide reliance on butter and salt ensures that no restaurant-prepared omelet will ever compare with one made in your own kitchen. But you can minimize fat with a meatless variety—thanks to the cheese, you still get an extra helping of protein.
500 calories, 29 g protein, 10 g carbs (2 g fiber, 4 g sugars), 37 g fat, 940 mg sodium

16. Best Egg-White Omelet
Bob Evans Western Omelet with Egg Whites
Fully half of the calories in this vegetable-packed omelet come from protein.
300 calories, 37 g protein, 6 g carbs (1 g fiber, 2 g sugars), 14 g fat, 1,364 mg sodium

17. Best Steak & Eggs
Bob Evans Sirloin Steak and Two Farm-Fresh Eggs
The best way to keep a steak-and-eggs breakfast under control is by going with a lean cut of meat—such as sirloin—and having it seared.
683 calories, 47 g protein, 5 g carbs (0 g fiber, 2 g sugars), 51 g fat, 1,096 mg sodium

18. Best Breakfast Potatoes
Bob Evans Home Fries (5.1 oz serving)
Bob's reign over the breakfast landscape is official. These are the least-greasy spuds you'll ever wake up to.
164 calories, 3 g protein, 24 g carbs (3 g fiber, 0 g sugars), 6 g fat, 680 mg sodium

MEXICAN

19. Best Drive-Thru Taco
Del Taco Chicken Taco Del Carbon (two tacos)
A double layer of warm corn tortillas wrapped around chicken, chili sauce, cilantro, and diced onions make these tacos the closest to the authentic Mexican version you'll ever buy from a drive-thru window.
300 calories, 18 g protein, 38 g carbs (2 g fiber, 2 g sugars), 10 g fat, 600 mg sodium

20. **Best Sit-Down Taco**

Baja Fresh Original Baja Chicken Tacos (two tacos)

Too many Mexican restaurants use inauthentic flour tortillas and pack on the cheese. But Baja Fresh sticks to basics: corn tortillas, chicken, onions, cilantro, and salsa.

420 calories, 24 g protein, 56 g carbs (4 g fiber, N/A sugars), 10 g fat, 460 mg sodium

21. **Best Fish Taco**

Baja Fresh Grilled Mahimahi

Most taco-bound seafood is battered and fried. Shed the crust of fat by sticking to this grilled option.

460 calories, 24 g protein, 52 g carbs (8 g fiber, N/A sugars), 18 g fat, 600 mg sodium

22. **Best Burrito**

Taco Bell Supreme Steak Fresco Burrito

Taco Bell promotes this burrito by touting the fact that it has less than 9 grams of fat, but far more impressive are the 16 grams of protein and 8 grams of fiber that they've managed to cram inside.

330 calories, 16 g protein, 50 g carbs (8 g fiber, 4 g sugars), 8 g fat, 1,340 mg sodium

23. **Best Fajitas**

On the Border Mesquite-Grilled Chicken with El Diablo veggies, guacamole, pico de gallo, and three flour tortillas

You're not going to find a low-calorie plate of fajitas, but you can temper the damage by skipping the cheese, sour cream, and rice, which will save you 450 calories. The sodium count is still high, though, so you may want to split this with your dinner partner.

825 calories, 54 g protein, 74 g carbs (4 g fiber, N/A g sugars), 35 g fat, 1,960 mg sodium

24. **Best Enchilada**

Chevys Salsa Chicken Enchiladas (two enchiladas)

Order these enchiladas à la carte with black beans on the side and you've just built one of the leanest entrees on Chevys menu.

460 calories, 30 g protein, 34 g carbs (4 g fiber, 6 g sugars), 22 g fat, 860 mg sodium

25. **Best Taquitos**

Taco Bell Grilled Steak Taquitos (two taquitos)

The classic taquito is cooked in a hot vat of oil, but Taco Bell gets the job done with a flattop grill. That means far fewer calories from fat.

310 calories, 15 g protein, 37 g carbs, (2 g fiber, 3 g sugars), 11 g fat, 930 mg sodium

26. **Best Quesadilla**
El Pollo Loco Cheese
Quesadilla
The same entrée at a sit-down restaurant will likely cost you more than 1,000 calories thanks to larger portion sizes and an excess of fillers.
420 calories, 19 g protein, 35 g carbs
(2 g fiber, 0 g sugars), 23 g fat,
810 mg sodium

27. **Best Nachos**
Taco Bell Triple-Layer Nachos
The generous helping of beans on these nachos leaves less room for cheese and brings in a commendable dose of fiber.
350 calories, 7 g protein, 39 g carbs
(7 g fiber, 2 g sugars), 18 g fat,
740 mg sodium

28. **Best Taco Salad**
Chipotle Barbacoa Salad Bowl
(lettuce, barbacoa, black
beans, guacamole, and green
tomatillo salsa; no vinaigrette)
By opting for guacamole and salsa instead of dressing, you add heart-healthy monounsaturated fats and a bevy of antioxidant-rich ingredients from the salsa.
465 calories, 35 g protein, 38 g carbs
(19 g fiber, 5 g sugars), 21 g fat,
1,185 mg sodium

29. **Best Tortilla Soup**
El Pollo Loco Regular Chicken
Tortilla Soup with Tortilla
Strips (10.8 oz)
Sodium is always an issue with tortilla soup, but El Pollo's recipe keeps the damage minimal while still supplying an impressive 16 grams of protein.
210 calories, 16 g protein, 18 g carbs
(2 g fiber, 2 g sugars), 9 g fat,
1,050 mg sodium

TRADITIONAL AMERICAN

30. **Best Steak**
Ruby Tuesday Plain-Grilled
Top Sirloin
Avoid the extra 1,000 milligrams of sodium that Ruby Tuesday uses to season the regular sirloin by ordering this 9-ounce steak "plain"—the restaurant's code word for "very little salt."
391 calories, 49 protein, 1 g carbs
(0 g fiber, N/A sugars), 22 g fat,
1,456 mg sodium

31. **Best Smothered Steak**
Applebee's 9-oz House Sirloin
Topped with Sautéed Garlic
Mushrooms
In restaurant-speak, "smothered" often means a jumble of greasy vegetables and a layer of cheese. Sautéed garlic and mushrooms are a much better option.
450 calories, 49 g protein, 1 g carbs
(0 g fiber, N/A sugars), 28 g fat,
1,190 mg sodium

32. **Best Ribs**
Ruby Tuesday Memphis Dry-Rub Fork-Tender Ribs (½ rack)
Leaner ribs simply cannot be found. At Outback Steakhouse, the half rack has nearly three times as much fat.
460 calories, 44 g protein, 6 g carbs (0 g fiber, N/A sugars), 29 g fat, 150 mg sodium

33. **Best Appetizer**
Ruby Tuesday Traditional Chicken Strips (four strips)
Being healthy doesn't mean skipping a starter. Just make sure you order these, which have the best nutritional profile around.
376 calories, N/A protein, 12 g carbs (0 g fiber, N/A sugars), 16 g fat, 888 mg sodium

34. **Best Chicken Entrée**
Olive Garden Venetian Apricot Chicken
Chicken and vegetables offer the perfect blend of protein and carbohydrates, and Olive Garden's tasty apricot citrus sauce is an extra bonus.
380 calories, N/A protein, 32 g carbs (8 g fiber, N/A sugars), 4 g fat, 1,420 mg sodium

35. **Best Barbecue Chicken**
Bob Evans Memphis Spice-Rubbed Chicken Breast
The Memphis-style rub—with ingredients such as garlic, onion, and cayenne pepper—is a great way to get that barbeque taste without loading up on calories and sodium.
281 calories, 30 g protein, 17 g carbs (1 g fiber, 15 g sugars), 10 g fat, 544 mg sodium

36. **Best Chicken Drumstick**
KFC Grilled Chicken Drumsticks (two drumsticks)
We know it's not called Kentucky Grilled Chicken, but choosing Grilled Drumsticks over KFC's Original Drumsticks will save you 100 calories and 7 grams of fat. Thanks, Colonel.
160 calories, 22 g protein, 0 g carbs, 8 g fat, 460 mg sodium

37. **Best Chicken Nuggets**
Chic-fil-A Nuggets (eight pieces)
Nugget for nugget, these chicken chunks have half as much fat as the McDonald's version.
270 calories, 28 g protein, 12 g carbs (1 g fiber, 2 g sugars), 12 g fat, 990 mg sodium

38. **Best Hot Dog**
Dairy Queen All-Beef Dog
When it comes to hot dogs, this one is as slim as they come. Practice prudence with the toppings and DQ's dog can be a fairly healthy protein-packed option.
290 calories, 11 g protein, 22 g carbs (1 g fiber, 4 g sugars), 17 g fat, 900 mg sodium

39. **Best Chili-Cheese Dog**
Dairy Queen All-Beef Chili-Cheese Dog
Consider this the most indulgent meal you'll ever find with fewer than 400 calories.
380 calories, 16 g protein, 23 g carbs (1 g fiber, 3 g sugars), 24 g fat, 980 mg sodium

40. Best Chili

Wendy's Chili (small)

With an ample amount of fiber and protein in tow, Wendy's chili is one of our all-time favorite fast-food sides. Choose it instead of medium fries and you'll save nearly 200 calories while gaining a boost of cancer-fighting lycopene.

220 calories, 18 g protein, 22 g carbs (6 g fiber, 6 g sugars), 7 g fat, 870 mg sodium

41. Best Bean Soup

Au Bon Pain Split-Pea-and-Ham (medium, 12 oz)

Fiber is a crucial element in the battle against unwanted weight gain, and this bowl of legumes has 50 percent of your day's recommended intake with a minor dose of fat.

250 calories, 18 g protein, 41 g carbs (15 g fiber, 3 g sugars), 2 g fat, 1,220 mg sodium

42. Best Chicken Noodle Soup

Applebee's Chicken Noodle Soup (bowl)

Commercially prepared soups are notoriously high in sodium, but at least this one boasts plenty of chicken to fill you up.

160 calories, 13 g protein, 17 g carbs (1 g fiber, N/A sugars), 4 g fat, 1,120 mg sodium

43. Best Cheesy Soup

Quiznos Broccoli-Cheese Soup (cup)

Some broccoli-and-cheese iterations are little more than a few florets floating in a sea of cheddar, so striking the proper balance between the two ingredients is crucial to your waistline. Just make sure you exercise portion control.

130 calories, 4 g protein, 9 g carbs (1 g fiber, 2 g sugars), 9 g fat, 640 mg sodium

44. Best Caesar Salad

California Pizza Kitchen Classic Caesar with Grilled Shrimp

Upgrading the classic recipe with shrimp is a great way to inject lean protein, selenium, and vitamin D into your meal.

649 calories, 35 g protein, 30 g carbs (8 g fiber, N/A sugars), 15 g saturated fat, 1,338 mg sodium

45. Best Fast-Food Meal

Chick-fil-A Chargrilled Chicken Sandwich with Large Fruit Cup

How do you build the world's best fast-food meal? Pair the best sandwich with a cup of nutrient-rich fruit. That's an entire meal with fewer calories than most medium orders of french fries.

400 calories, 30 g protein, 65 g carbs (6 g fiber, 32 g sugars), 3.5 g fat, 1,120 mg sodium

46. Best Fast-Food Side

Taco Bell Pintos 'N Cheese
The pinto beans in this cup happen to be one of the planet's healthiest foods. They're rich in fiber, antioxidants, and folate, a B vitamin with a strong link to weight loss. We'll take these over nachos any day.
170 calories, 10 g protein, 19 g carbs (9 g fiber, 1 g sugars), 6 g fat, 750 mg sodium

BURGERS AND SANDWICHES

47. Best Fast-Food Burger

McDonald's Big N' Tasty (no mayo)
Ordered sans mayo, the Big N' Tasty is without a doubt the leanest fast-food burger of its size.
410 calories, 24 g protein, 36 g carbs (3 g fiber, 7 g sugars), 19 g fat, 640 mg sodium

48. Best Sit-Down Restaurant Burger

Red Robin Natural Burger
Most burgers have been embellished so much that they're barely recognizable beneath the excess layers of fat. This is one of the few that keeps it simple, clocking in under 600 calories.
569 calories, 37 g protein, 51 g carbs (3 g fiber, 9 g sugars), 24 g fat, 989 mg sodium

49. Best Mushroom Burger

Culver's Mushroom & Swiss Single
The law of burgers states that the longer the name, the worse the burger is for you. This one's an exception to the rule.
431 calories, 25 g protein, 33 g carbs (1 g fiber, 5 g sugars), 20 g fat, 581 mg sodium

50. Best Bacon Burger

Five Guys Little Bacon Burger
"Little" this burger most certainly is not, but to the folks at Five Guys, anything bigger than "little" amounts to a double burger. So take the little single—it's the biggest bacon burger you'll find under 600 calories.
560 calories, 27 g protein, 39 g carbs (2 g fiber, 8 g sugars), 33 g fat, 640 mg sodium

51. Best Double Burger

Wendy's Double Stack
Thanks to a double portion of Wendy's Jr. patties, this burger keeps the calories low but the meat-to-bun ratio high.
360 calories, 23 g protein, 27 g carbs (1 g fiber, 6 g sugars), 18 g fat, 760 mg sodium

52. **Best Turkey Burger**
Red Robin Grilled
Turkey Burger
Turkey burgers are generally no healthier than their beef-based counterparts. (Many restaurants use fattier turkey for a juicier burger.) Order one at Ruby Tuesday, for instance, and you're risking a 1,230-calorie backlash. This one's much more reasonable.
641 calories, 30 g protein, 50 g carbs
(3 g fiber, 8 g sugars), 37 g fat,
1,000 mg sodium

53. **Best Veggie Burger**
Burger King BK Veggie Burger
Of the big-three fast-food purveyors, Burger King is the only one that offers a veggie burger. And great news for busy vegetarians: It trounces the veggie offerings from all the major sit-and-eat chains.
400 calories, 22 g protein, 43 g carbs
(N/A fiber, 8 g sugars), 16 g fat,
1,020 mg sodium

54. **Best French Fries**
McDonald's French Fries
(medium)
You can find lower-calorie fries at KFC and Dairy Queen, but both chains still rely on partially hydrogenated oils to crisp their spuds. Plus McD's fries have less than half as much sodium.
380 calories, 4 g protein, 48 g carbs
(5 g fiber, 0 g sugars), 19 g fat,
270 mg sodium

55. **Best Fried Onion**
Burger King Onion Rings
(small)
The lowest-calorie rings we could find. Plus Burger King uses vegetable oil rather than trans-fatty partially hydrogenated oil.
310 calories, 4 g protein, 36 g carbs
(3 g fiber, 4 g sugars), 17 g fat,
490 mg sodium

56. **Best Chicken Wings**
Pizza Hut WingStreet
All-American
Traditional Wings
(five wings)
Hands down the lightest recipe when it comes to wings. Just make sure you order them "traditional" style. Ask for it "crispy" and you can expect nearly three times the fat.
400 calories, 35 g protein, 0 g carbs,
25 g fat, 1,450 mg sodium

57. **Best Roast Beef Sandwich**
Subway Roast Beef Sub
(6-inch on 9-grain wheat
bread)
Not only is this sandwich leaner than any of the roast-beef offerings at Arby's but you can also load it up with healthy vegetables.
310 calories, 26 g protein, 45 g carbs
(5 g fiber, 6 g sugars), 4.5 g fat,
800 mg sodium

58. **Best Steak Sandwich**

Quiznos Roadhouse
Steak Sammie

The bread used in the sammie is smaller than typical sandwich bread, which means more calories to spend on sautéed mushrooms, onions, and Quiznos' Sweet and Spicy Steak Sauce.

260 calories, 13 g protein, 38 g carbs (1 g fiber, 13 g sugars), 6 g fat, 980 mg sodium

59. **Best BLT**

Five Guys BLT (4 slices of bacon, lettuce, tomato, and mustard)

Even if you don't see a BLT on the menu, burger joints are equipped to put them together. Build your own at Five Guys and it'll be leaner than any burger the chain has to offer.

433 calories, 24 g protein, 42 g carbs (3 g fiber, 11 g sugars), 23 g fat, 911 mg sodium

60. **Best Reuben**

Schlotzsky's Small Angus Pastrami Reuben

The classic Reuben relies on a fat-packed triad of Thousand Island dressing, Swiss cheese, and corned beef. This version is the healthiest one you'll find with those ingredients.

618 calories, 41 g protein, 54 g carbs (4 g fiber, 4 g sugars), 26 g fat, 1,510 mg sodium

60. **Best Pulled Pork Sandwich**

White Castle Pulled Pork BBQ Sandwich (2)

This is as close to guilt-free as you can get with a pulled-pork BBQ sandwich. Even having three would be better than any other restaurant option.

340 calories, 18 g protein, 50 g carbs, (2 g fiber, 24 g sugars), 9 g fat, 920 mg sodium

62. **Best Ham and Cheese Sandwich**

Arby's Ham & Swiss Melt Sandwich

This warm, toasty sandwich satisfies despite its modest size.

300 calories, 18 g protein, 37 g carbs (2 g fiber, 6 g sugars), 8 g fat, 1,070 mg sodium

63. **Best Mini Sandwiches**

KFC Honey BBQ Snackers (two sandwiches)

For comparison, White Castle's healthiest chicken sandwich carries an extra 140 calories.

420 calories, 26 g protein, 64 g carbs (4 g fiber, 24 g sugars), 6 g fat, 940 mg sodium

64. **Best Grilled Chicken Sandwich**

Chic-fil-A Char-Grilled Chicken Sandwich

Low in calories and high in protein, this sandwich is one of the fast-food world's greatest achievements. Pair it with a fruit cup for a perfectly rounded lunch.

300 calories, 29 g protein, 38 g carbs (3 g fiber, 10 g sugars), 3.5 g fat, 1,120 mg sodium

65. Best Crispy Chicken Sandwich

Wendy's Crispy
Chicken Sandwich

Wendy's manages what no other fast food joint has been able to: Make a crispy chicken sandwich with fewer than 400 calories and less than 1,000 milligrams of sodium.

350 calories, 15 g protein, 38 g carbs
(2 g fiber, 4 g sugars), 15 g fat,
830 g sodium

66. Best Chicken Salad Sandwich

Atlanta Bread Company
Chicken Salad on Sourdough

ABC's recipe bucks bad restaurant habits by maintaining the proper ratio of chicken to mayonnaise.

440 calories, 29 g protein, 42 g carbs
(3 g fiber, 4 g sugars), 19 g fat,
680 mg sodium

67. Best Classic Fish Sandwich

McDonald's Filet-O-Fish

There are two ingredients that, when applied carelessly, can overpower the fish and sink the nutritional value: cheese and tartar sauce. Thankfully, McDonald's applies both with due prudence.

380 calories, 15 g protein, 38 g carbs
(2 g fiber, 5 g sugars), 18 g fat,
640 mg sodium

68. Best Melt

Arby's Melt

Arby's roast beef has a peppery tang that pairs perfectly with the mellow flavor of Cheddar cheese. And it's leaner than a burger.

370 calories, 23 g protein, 40 g carbs
(2 g fiber, 6 g sugars), 13 g fat,
1,150 mg sodium

69. Best Philly Cheesesteak

Subway Big Philly Cheesesteak (6-inch on 9-grain whole wheat)

The sheer amount of beef makes this one of the most filling sandwiches on Subway's menu. And, thankfully, it relies on real cheese instead of Cheez Whiz.

520 calories, 39 g protein, 53 g carbs
(6 g fiber, 7 g sugars), 18 g fat,
1,570 mg sodium

70. Best Veggie Sandwich

Cosi Fire-Roasted
Veggie Sandwich

Finally, there's a veggie sandwich that's more than just a garden salad between two pieces of bread. To deliver big flavor, Cosi brings in eggplant, roasted peppers, artichoke hearts, hummus, and feta, which helps bolster the protein count, too.

324 calories, 11 g protein, 44 g carbs
(4 g fiber, 4 g sugars), 8 g fat,
259 mg sodium

71. **Best Wrap**
Dairy Queen Grilled Chicken Wrap

Few restaurants seem able to make a chicken wrap without injecting a turkey baster's worth of mayonnaise. DQ manages otherwise. Sure, there's a touch of ranch sauce in this wrap, but it still adds up to a low calorie count.

200 calories, 12 g protein, 9 g carbs (1 g fiber, 1 g sugars), 13 g fat, 450 mg sodium

ASIAN

72. **Best Dumplings**
P.F. Chang's Steamed Pork Dumplings (six dumplings)

Ask for them steamed instead of pan-fried and cut 2 grams of fat from each dumpling.

360 calories, 24 g protein, 36 g carbs (0 g fiber, N/A sugars), 12 g fat, 750 mg sodium

73. **Best (two) Chinese Entrées**
Manchu Wok Beef and Broccoli with Green Bean Chicken

The best Chinese entrée is actually two! But only if you order strategically. The usual approach at Chinese restaurants is to burden each plate with 300 to 450 calories of pure starch via noodles or rice. Skip those carbo-bombs and calories by ordering these two balanced entrées à la carte.

340 calories, 15 g protein, 22 g carbs (4 g fiber, 8 g sugars), 23 g fat, 1,290 mg sodium

74. **Best Spicy Dish**
Panda Express Kung Pao Chicken with Mixed Veggies

Kung Pao's peanuts deliver a nice package of metabolism-boosting B vitamins, and the mixed veggies sneak in some fiber, as well.

335 calories, 21 g protein, 21 g carbs (5 g fiber, 6 g sugars), 19 g fat, 1,140 mg sodium

75. **Best Pork Dish**
Manchu Wok BBQ Pork with Mixed Vegetables

Pick this dish next time you need a dose of Chinese-style pork. The sweet-and-sour version carries more sugar and less protein.

370 calories, 24 g protein, 27 g carbs (3 g fiber, 16 g sugars), 21 g fat, 1,240 mg sodium

76. **Best Side**
P.F. Chang's Spinach Stir-Fried with Garlic (small)

We always recommend replacing rice and chow mein with more rewarding ingredients, but rarely does Asian cuisine present the opportunity to enjoy vitamin-rich spinach with your meal.

80 calories, 6 g protein, 7.5 g carbs (4.5 g fiber, N/A sugars), 4.5 g fat, 450 mg sodium

77. **Best Spring Roll/or Egg Roll**
Manchu Wok Chicken
Egg Roll (one roll)
With egg rolls, it's all about portion control. These deep-fried torpedoes can sink your chance of a healthy meal, so stick with just one and keep it around 150 calories.
150 calories, 5 g protein, 17 g carbs (1 g fiber, 1 g sugars), 7 g fat, 350 mg sodium

78. **Best Asian Soup**
Panda Express Egg
Flower Soup
This bowl manages two rare feats in the soup world: It carries fewer than 100 calories and has less than 1,000 milligrams of sodium.
90 calories, 3 g protein, 15 g carbs (1 g fiber, 4 g sugars), 2 g fat, 810 mg sodium

79. **Best Asian Salad**
Panera Asian Sesame
Chicken Salad
Most Asian salads suffer from an overload of either sugar or sodium. Panera's avoids both while emphasizing lean protein.
400 calories, 31 g protein, 31 g carbs (3 g fiber, 6 g sugars), 20 g fat, 810 mg sodium

ITALIAN

80. **Best Spaghetti**
Fazoli's Spaghetti or
Penne Marinara
A modest amount of fat and antioxidant-packed tomatoes make marinara the best sauce for any pasta dish.
560 calories, 19 g protein, 111 carbs (9 g fiber, 17 g sugars), 2.5 g fat, 970 mg sodium

81. **Best Alfredo**
Red Lobster Crab Linguine
Alfredo (lunch portion)
Made from butter, Parmesan cheese, and cream, Alfredo drowns pasta in excess fat and sodium. Halve your portion, toss in some protein for good measure, and that's a meal well managed.
560 calories, N/A protein, 47 g carbs (N/A fiber, N/A sugars), 25 g fat, 1,310 mg sodium

82. **Best Stuffed Pasta**
Olive Garden's Ravioli di
Portobello (lunch portion)
Low in sodium and a great source of fiber, portobello mushrooms are a delicious—and smart—way to fill your ravioli and you.
450 calories, N/A protein, 53 g carbs (8 g fiber, N/A sugars), 19 g fat, 960 mg sodium

83. **Best Chicken Pasta**
Fazoli's Penne with Marinara, Broccoli, and Sliced Grilled Chicken

Fazoli's might be the fast food of Italian cuisine, but it's also the place that gives you the most control over your entrée. Keep it simple with a combo like this and you'll be better off.

695 calories, 39 g protein, 118 mg carbs (12 g fiber, 19 g sugars), 6 g fat, 1,490 mg sodium

84. **Best Lasagna**
Olive Garden's Lasagna Classico (lunch portion)

The full portion of this meal contains 2,830 milligrams of sodium and roughly one-third of your daily caloric intake. Lunch portions are an easy way to satisfy your craving without chaining you to the treadmill.

580 calories, N/A protein, 35 g carbs (7 g fiber, N/A sugars), 32 g fat, 1,930 mg sodium

85. **Best Parmesan**
Olive Garden Eggplant Parmigiana

The word "parmigiana" on a menu usually means trouble, but if you must, eggplant is a good source of fiber and will always save you calories over heavier options such as veal or chicken. Add a side of broccoli—the potassium will help balance the high sodium count.

850 calories, 98 g carbs (19 g fiber), 35 g fat, 1,900 mg sodium

86. **Best Italian Soup**
Culver's Minestrone (300 g)

Minestrone ingredients vary, but you can always depend on a bowl chock-full of vegetables, which keep the calorie count low while providing plenty of flavor and fiber.

100 calories, 4 g protein, 19 g carbs (4 g fiber, 4 g sugars), 1 g fat, 1,175 mg sodium

87. **Best Pizza**
Pizza Hut 12" Fit and Delicious, with Chicken, Mushrooms, and Jalapeño (two slices)

The Hut's Fit and Delicious line is by far the healthiest choice at any of the major pizza chains. Chicken, mushrooms, and jalapeños layer each slice with protein, a bit of fiber, and a touch of heat. Just make sure you exercise some discipline and stick to two slices.

340 calories, 22 g protein, 44 g carbs (2 g fiber, 8 g sugars), 9 g fat, 1,440 mg sodium

88. **Best Personal Pizza**
Pizza Hut Pepperoni and Mushroom Personal Pan Pizza

In this case, toppings are a good thing: Surprisingly, the plain cheese version has 20 extra calories.

570 calories, 24 g protein, 68 g carbs (4 g fiber, 7 g sugars), 23 g fat, 1,250 mg sodium

89. Best Vegetarian Pizza

Pizza Hut 12" Fit and Delicious, with Green Peppers, Red Onion, and Diced Red Tomato (two slices)

You save 100 calories compared to two slices of Pizza Hut's 12" Hand-Tossed Veggie Lover's.

300 calories, 12 g protein, 48 g carbs (4 g fiber, 10 g sugars), 8 g fat, 800 mg sodium

90. Best Flatbread

Uno Chicago Grill Roasted Eggplant, Spinach, and Feta (½ flatbread)

The feta's fat load is balanced with a heavy hit of protein. Spinach and eggplant only bring good energy to this party, so fret not and enjoy.

510 calories, 27 g protein, 58.5 g carbs (1.5 g fiber, 13.5 g sugars), 13 g fat, 990 mg sodium

SEAFOOD

91. Best Seafood Appetizer

Outback Seared Ahi Tuna (small)

When it comes to appetizers—especially at Outback—this plate of protein is a great way to start any meal. Just don't go overboard with the creamy ginger soy sauce and wasabi vinaigrette dipping sauces.

355 calories, 18.3 g protein, 11.5 g carbs (2.2 g fiber), 23.3 g fat, 1,660 mg sodium

92. Best Fish Filet Entrée

Red Lobster Blackened Salmon with Broccoli

Salmon has an abundance of omega-3s, which have been shown to reduce your risk of heart disease. And since the fish isn't smothered in creamy sauce, the entrée is still low in fat.

490 calories, 6 g carbs, 17 g fat, 440 mg sodium

93. Best Shrimp Entrée

Houlihan's Grilled Shrimp Entrée with Panzanella Bread Salad and Grilled Asparagus

Shrimp is low in saturated fat and high in protein—as long as it avoids the deep fryer and fat-packed sauces.

556 calories, 48 protein, 32 g carbs, (5 g fiber), 26 g fat, 1,239 mg sodium

94. Best Breaded Fish

Red Lobster Fried Flounder

Fish is a dish best served plain, but if you prefer it fried, avoid the trans fat by making sure the restaurant doesn't use partially hydrogenated oil. A light flaky fish such as flounder will also help keep the calorie count to a minimum.

440 calories, N/A g protein, 5 g carbs, 16 g fat, 560 mg sodium

95. Best Crab Cakes

Long John Silver's Langostino Lobster-Stuffed Crab Cake

These decadent-sounding crab cakes pack in plenty of seafood but still boast a low calorie count.

170 calories, 6 g protein, 1 g fiber, 9 g fat, 390 mg sodium

96. Best Shrimp Appetizer

Red Lobster Chilled Jumbo
Shrimp Cocktail

*You'd be hard-pressed to find
another appetizer that gives you this
much protein for so few calories.
Plus, shrimp is a great source of
selenium, an antioxidant that may
help prevent cancer.*

120 calories, N/A g protein, 9 g carbs
(N/A g fiber, N/A g sugars), 0.5 g fat,
580 mg sodium

97. Best Clam Chowder

Subway New England Clam
Chowder (10-oz bowl)

*Plenty of New England–style clam
chowders are heavy, but that isn't a
problem at Subway.*

150 calories, 6 g protein, 20 g carbs
(4 g fiber, 2 g sugars), 5 g fat, 990 mg
sodium

98. Best Surf and Turf

Red Lobster Wood-Grilled
Peppercorn Sirloin with
Steamed Snow Crab Legs

*If you want to eat by land and by sea,
snow crab legs and a modest portion of
lean grilled steak are a great pair. The
sodium count is high, though, so avoid
the salt shaker for the rest of the day.*

360 calories, N/A g protein, 0 g carbs,
10.5 g fat, 1,790 mg sodium

99. Best Seafood Salad

Macaroni Grill Scallops and
Spinach Salad

*Seared scallops will fill you up,
and the fresh, wilted spinach provides
a bevy of nutrients. Ask them to
leave out the prosciutto to lower
the sodium.*

340 calories, 8 g protein, 11 g carbs
(4 g fiber, N/A sugars), 31 g fat,
820 mg sodium

DESSERT

100. Best Ice Cream

Ben & Jerry's Scoop Shop
Coffee Ice Cream (one scoop)

*Just one scoop of ice cream can be a
sugar land mine, especially when it's
packed with swirls and bits of candy.
This Ben & Jerry's flavor keeps the
calories and sugar in check without
being plain ol' vanilla.*

190 calories, 3 g protein, 18 g carbs
(0 g fiber, 16 g sugars), 11 g fat,
50 mg sodium

101. Best Ice Cream Novelty

Dairy Queen Ice
Cream Sandwich

*Somehow DQ has sandwiched ice
cream between two chocolate wafers
and made a treat that is no worse
than a single scoop of ice cream. Don't
ask questions; just be thankful.*

190 calories, 4 g protein, 31 g carbs
(1 g fiber, 18 g sugars), 5 g fat

102. Best Ice Cream Topping

Cold Stone Creamery
Blueberries (15 g)

*Blueberries are packed with antioxi-
dants – and an intense hit of flavor.
And since Cold Stone Creamery offers
them as a healthy mix-in option,
there's absolutely no need to add
candy bar chunks to your ice cream.*

10 calories, 0 g protein, 2 g carbs
(0 g fiber, 2 g sugars), 0 g fat

103. Best Frozen Yogurt
Ben & Jerry's Vanilla Low-Fat
Frozen Yogurt (one scoop)
Frozen yogurt carries less fat than ice cream, but to compensate, processors often jack up the sugar levels. This version is just the balance you're looking for.
130 calories, 4 g protein, 25 g carbs
(0 g fiber, 16 g sugar), 1.5 g fat,
70 mg sodium

104. Best Sorbet
Macaroni Grill Italian Sorbetto
Made with lemons and raspberries, this dessert is a cool way to get your vitamin C fix.
150 calories, 0 g protein, 37 g carbs
(0 g fiber, N/A sugars), 0 g fat,
5 mg sodium

105. Best Ice
Culver's Lemon Ice
(one scoop)
Ice and flavored syrup are all that goes into this summer-day salvation with a surprisingly modest amount of sugar.
84 calories, 0 g protein, 21 g carbs
(0 g fiber, 18 g sugars), 0 g fat,
4 g sodium

106. Best Root Beer Float
A&W Root Beer Float
(small, 16 oz)
No one does root beer better than A&W, and the same goes for floats. Ruby Tuesday's float, by comparison, has 169 extra calories and almost three times as much fat.
330 calories, 2 g protein, 70 g carbs
(0 g fiber, 57 g sugars), 5 g fat,
100 mg sodium

107. Best Sundae
Uno Chicago Grill Mini
Bananas Foster (168 g)
Sure, there are sundaes with less fat and sugar, but do they come drizzled with a dose of rum? Nope. And since the portion size is under control, it's a smart indulgence.
350 calories, 4 g protein, 46 g carbs
(1 g fiber, 36 g sugars), 17 g fat,
140 mg sodium

108. Best Brownie Sundae
Uno Chicago Grill Mini Hot
Chocolate Brownie Sundae
A brownie sundae is basically two desserts in one. Uno's mini portion lets you enjoy the combo while avoiding a calorie crisis.
370 calories, 4 g protein, 54 g carbs
(2 g fiber, 38 g sugars), 16 g fat,
1950 mg sodium

109. Best Banana Split
Sonic's Junior Banana Split
(134 g)
Do you really need three helpings of ice cream in your banana split? Of course not. This one governs the heavy scooping and provides a dose of banana-based potassium.
210 calories, 2 g protein, 37 g carbs
(1 g fiber, 26 g sugars), 6 g fat,
90 mg sodium

110. **Best Cheesecake**

Schlotzky's New York–Style
Cheesecake (one slice)
Packed with cream cheese, cheese-cake is often described as sinfully good, but a sinner you don't have to be. This slice from Schlotzky's has 315 fewer calories and 12 grams less satu-rated fat than Cheesecake Factory's Original Cheesecake.
350 calories, 6 g protein, 30 g carbs
(1 g fiber, 19 g sugars), 23 g fat,
200 mg sodium

111. **Best Chocolate Cake**

Jack in the Box Chocolate
Overload Cake (one slice)
An intense hit of chocolate doesn't mean a mandatory overload of calories and fat. You'd be hard-pressed to find a better deal than this quick treat.
300 calories, 4 g protein, 57 g carbs
(2 g fiber, 34 g sugars), 7 g fat,
350 mg sodium

112. **Best Apple Pie**

McDonald's Baked
Hot Apple Pie
More of a pocket than a traditional apple pie, but it's tasty and carries a modest amount of calories compared with other versions.
250 calories, 2 g protein, 32 g carbs
(4 g fiber, 13 g sugars), 13 g fat,
170 mg sodium

113. **Best Key Lime Pie**

Chili's Sweet Shot
Key Lime Pie
Served in a shot glass, this is a great alternative to ordering a whole slice. Calories will add up fast if you get a Sweet Shot Sampler, though, so resist the urge.
240 calories, 4 g protein, 30 g carbs
(0 g fiber, N/A sugars), 12 g fat,
75 mg sodium

DRINKS

114. **Best Coffee**

McDonald's Premium
Roast (small, 12 oz)
The confines of the dollar menu keep it cheap, and the special blend of Arabica beans keeps it rich. It's just how a cup of joe should be.
0 calories

115. **Best Espresso Drink**

Starbucks Cappuccino with
2 Percent Milk (grande, 16 oz)
Choices abound at any coffee shop, but the "simpler is better" mantra applies here, too. A cappuccino contains more froth and less fluid milk than a latte, which means fewer calories.
120 calories, 8 g protein, 12 g carbs
(0 g fiber, 10 g sugar), 4 g fat,
85 mg sodium

116. Best Iced Coffee Drink

Starbuck's Grande Iced Caffe Americano (grande, 16 oz)

Starbuck's Iced Americano is just a shot of espresso diluted with water and served over ice, providing a naturally subtle sweetness that encourages a more sophisticated coffee palate.

15 calories, <1 protein, 3 g carbs (0 g fiber, 0 g sugars), 0 g fat, 10 mg sodium

117. Best Blended Coffee Drink

Smoothie King Skinny Coffee Smoothie Mocha (small, 20 oz)

Protein powder and nonfat milk make this by far the best blended coffee drink available.

260 calories, 17 g protein, 43 carbs (1 g fiber, 36 g sugars), 2 g fat, 226 mg sodium

118. Best Hot Tea

Jamba Juice Mighty Tea Leaf Organic Green Dragon Tea (16 oz)

Mighty Leaf uses premium green tea from China and their roomy tea bags allow the leaves to fully unfold, maximizing the infusion process.

0 calories

119. Best Sweetened Tea Drink

Starbucks Tazo Shaken Iced Green Tea (grande, 16 oz)

Specialty green tea drinks are all the rage, but the best ones give you a dose of antioxidants without an excess of sugar. This Starbucks drink does the trick.

80 calories, 0 g protein, 21 g carbs (0 g fiber, 20 g sugars), 0 g fat, 10 mg sodium

120. Best Fruit Smoothie

Smoothie King Blueberry Heaven (small, 20 oz)

Like most smoothies, this version is relatively high in sugar, but it redeems itself with a helping of protein and fiber. Just don't go for the jumbo size.

325 calories, 7 g protein, 73 g carbs (2 g fiber, 64 g sugar), 1 g fat, 259 mg sodium

121. Best Protein Smoothie

Smoothie King High-Protein Banana (20 oz)

This smoothie is a great meal replacer, low in calories but high in protein. It also contains almonds, which augment the protein count while also offering heart-healthy monounsaturated fats.

322 calories, 27 g protein, 32 g carbs (4 g fiber, 23 g sugar), 9 g fat, 297 mg sodium

122. **Best Slush**

Sonic's Lemon Real Fruit Slush (medium, 20 oz)

Typically, slushes are a mixture of ice and sugar-laden syrup. Sonic's gets credit for bringing i n a touch of real fruit.

290 calories, 0 g protein, 78 g carbs (0 g fiber, 74 g sugars), 0 g fat, 45 mg sodium

123. **Best Cocktail**

Red Lobster Rob Roy

Cocktails often include several sugary mixers with an already sweet liqueur. A Rob Roy keeps it simple with scotch and sweet vermouth. Ask for the drink with dry vermouth to minimize your sugar intake.

160 calories, N/A protein, 3 g carbs (N/A fiber, N/A sugars), 0 g fat, 10 mg sodium

124. **Best Margarita**

Olive Garden Wild Berry Frozen Margarita

The rare frozen margarita under 300 calories.

290 calories, N/A g protein 55 g carbs, (N/A g fiber, N/A g sugar) 0 g fat, 20 mg sodium

125. **Best Juice**

Jamba Juice Carrot Juice (12 oz)

A 12-ounce serving of this juice pro- vides 700 percent of your day's vita- min A requirement plus shots of both vitamin C and calcium in the same number of calories as you'd find in 8 ounces of Pepsi. The Pepsi, however, scores nil for nutrients.

100 calories, 3 g protein, 22 carbs (0 g fiber, 20 g sugars), 0.5 g fat, 170 mg sodium

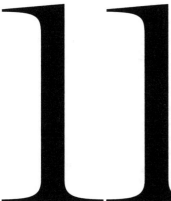

THE *WOMEN'S HEALTH* DIET RECIPES
Mouthwatering concoctions to keep you full and to fight fat

The *Women's Health* Diet is designed to melt away pounds, not by cutting down on the amount of food you eat, but by filling you with nutrient-rich meals and snacks that are satisfying and delicious. By following the *Women's Health* Secrets of the Slim, you'll strip away fat and useless calories along with the unhealthy, artificial compounds found in many processed foods that have been shown to contribute to weight gain.

The following recipes are quick and easy to follow. They'll help you stick to the Secrets of the Slim, because you'll stay full all day long as you burn calories easily and naturally—even while you sleep! And you'll feel healthier and happier, because *The Women's Health Diet* is designed to boost not only your body's fat-burning furnace but your brain's natural mood stabilizers, as well.

The *Women's Health* Diet Breakfasts

Focus on eating a lot of calories in the form of dairy, eggs, whole grains, and fiber

When you shift calories to the morning, you lose weight and keep it off. So eat a large portion of your daily calories—30 to 35 percent of your total intake—in the morning. If you usually skip breakfast, you'll discover that you'll actually eat fewer calories throughout the day and gain less weight simply by eating two eggs and a slice of whole-grain toast every morning. And if you have neither the time nor the stomach for a big breakfast first thing in the morning, try having two breakfasts—something small right after you get up, like a glass of milk and whole-wheat toast, and a larger breakfast or snack an hour or so later.

Spinach and Smoked Salmon Breakfast Burrito

2 Tbsp ricotta cheese

1 medium whole-wheat tortilla

1 oz smoked salmon, torn into little pieces

2 eggs, scrambled in a non-stick pan

1 cup baby spinach, chopped

1 green onion, sliced

Spread the cheese on the tortilla, then arrange the salmon, eggs, spinach, and green onions on top. Fold the ends in, roll, and enjoy.

Makes 1 serving. Per serving: *372 calories, 38 g protein, 25 g carbs, 3 g fiber, 2 g sugars, 16 g fat, 477 mg cholesterol, 392 mg sodium*

Vegetable Garden Omelet

5 large eggs

half a fistful of fresh parsley, chopped

splash of soy sauce

2 tsp olive oil

2 Tbsp broccoli florets

5 spears asparagus, chopped

¼ cup string beans, halved

½ cup spinach

1 clove garlic, chopped

dash of black pepper

1. Mix the eggs, parsley, and soy sauce in a bowl.

2. Coat a skillet with the olive oil and sauté the broccoli, asparagus, beans, spinach, garlic, and black pepper for 5 minutes.

3. Pour the egg mixture over the vegetables. Stir it for about 30 seconds and then let it sit for 1 minute. Stir it again until the eggs firm up and then let it sit for another minute. Then fold it and remove it from the pan.

Makes 2 servings. Per serving: *223 calories, 15 g protein, 5 g carbs, 2 g fiber, 3 g sugars, 14 g fat, 525 mg cholesterol, 172 mg sodium*

Berry Walnut Quinoa

1 cup quinoa, rinsed
2 cups apple juice
¼ cup walnuts, crushed
1 cup organic berries
   dash of cinnamon
3 mint leaves

1. In a saucepan, bring the quinoa and apple juice to a boil and then lower the heat to a simmer.

2. Cover and cook for 15 minutes until the quinoa is translucent.

3. Remove the pan from the heat and let the quinoa rest, covered, for 2 minutes. Put it into a bowl and stir in the nuts, berries, cinnamon, and mint.

Makes 2 servings. Per serving: *367 calories, 7 g protein, 62 g carbs, 6 g fiber, 35 g sugars, 12 g fat, 0 mg cholesterol, 15 mg sodium*

Cranberry Walnut Porridge

½ cup evaporated milk
2 Tbsp whole-grain Cream of Wheat cereal or Wheatena
1 Tbsp flaxseed, ground
½ tsp vanilla extract
1 Tbsp walnuts, chopped
1 tsp maple syrup
1 Tbsp dried cranberries

1. Combine the milk and cereal in a microwaveable bowl or mixing cup. Whisk with a fork. Microwave on high power for 2 minutes. Whisk again. Microwave in 30-second intervals, whisking after each interval, for about 60 seconds or until thickened. Stir in the flaxseed and vanilla extract. Spoon into a cereal bowl. Set aside.

2. Coat a small microwaveable plate with cooking spray. Spread the walnuts on the plate. Drizzle them with syrup. Microwave on high power for about 45 seconds or until sizzling. Using a spatula, scatter the glazed walnuts over the cereal mixture. Top with the cranberries.

Makes 1 serving. Per serving: *370 calories, 14 g protein, 44 g carbs, 5 g fiber, 21 g sugars, 16 g fat, 35 mg cholesterol, 140 mg sodium*

Tortillas with Spinach, Black Beans, and Cheddar

5 soft corn tortillas (6" diameter)

6 scallions, chopped

1 red bell pepper, chopped

1 small jalapeño pepper, seeded and finely chopped (optional)

1 clove garlic, minced

1 tsp ground cumin

1 can (15 oz) reduced-sodium black beans, rinsed and drained

4 cups (about 4 oz) baby spinach

1 large tomato, chopped

1 cup Cheddar cheese, shredded

4 Tbsp sour cream

fresh cilantro, chopped, for garnish

1. Preheat the oven to 350°F. Stack the tortillas on a large piece of foil, sprinkle the top one with water, and wrap them in the foil. Heat for 10 minutes.

2. Meanwhile, heat a large skillet coated with olive oil cooking spray over medium-high heat. Add the scallions and bell pepper and cook for 5 minutes, or until lightly browned. Add the jalapeño pepper (if using), garlic, and cumin. Cook for 2 minutes or until lightly browned. Stir in the beans, spinach, and tomato. Cook for 2 minutes or until heated through. Spread the mixture evenly in the skillet.

3. Remove the mixture from the heat and sprinkle it with the cheese. Let it stand until the cheese is melted. Top with dollops of sour cream and sprinkle it with the cilantro.

4. Cut the warmed tortillas into quarters or strips. Serve immediately with the cheesy bean-vegetable mixture.

Makes 4 servings. Per serving: *275 calories, 14 g protein, 30 g carbs, 9 g fiber, 4 g sugars, 13 g fat, 35 mg cholesterol, 446 mg sodium*

Egg Sandwich with Spinach, Bacon, and Cheese

1   slice (1 oz) bacon
½   tsp extra-virgin olive oil
1   egg
1   multigrain English muffin, toasted
1½   oz (about 1 cup, packed) trimmed spinach leaves or baby spinach
    freshly ground black pepper
1   slice Swiss, Jarlsberg, or Havarti cheese

1. Cook bacon slice per package directions.

2. Heat the oil in a small skillet over medium heat. Add the egg and heat it until the edges begin to set, about 1 minute. Lift the edges to allow any uncooked egg to flow underneath. When it's almost set, gently flip the egg. Cook another minute, then transfer to the bottom half of the muffin and top with the bacon.

3. Return the pan to the heat, add the spinach, and cook, stirring until it's wilted, about 1 minute. Place the spinach on top of the bacon, season with the pepper, add the cheese, and top with the other muffin half.

Makes 1 serving. Per serving (with Swiss cheese): *270 g calories, 20 g protein, 28 g carbs, 6 g fiber, 2 g sugars, 14 g fat, 20 mg cholesterol, 200 mg sodium*

Veggie Frittata Pocket

4   white mushrooms, sliced
1   Tbsp onion, chopped
1   Tbsp red bell pepper, chopped
    pinch of ground black pepper
2   eggs
½   small tomato, seeded and chopped
3   Tbsp milk
1   whole-wheat pita, halved and toasted
½   avocado, sliced

1. Coat a skillet with olive oil cooking spray and place over medium heat. Add the mushrooms, onion, bell pepper, and black pepper. Cook for 3 to 4 minutes.

2. Meanwhile, in a bowl, combine the eggs, tomato, and milk. Whisk together until frothy. Pour the egg mixture into the skillet. Cook, stirring, for 3 to 4 minutes, or until the eggs are firm.

3. Fill each pita with half the eggs and top with the avocado slices.

Makes 1 serving. Per serving: *436 calories, 22 g protein, 40 g carbs, 9 g fiber, 7 g sugars, 23 g fat, 428 mg cholesterol, 411 mg sodium,*

Oven-Roasted Oats
with Fruit and Sunflower Seeds

6 cups old-fashioned oats, preferably thick-cut

1¼ cups raw almonds, sliced

1 package (7 oz) dried fruit bits

1 cup toasted wheat germ

½ cup unsalted raw pumpkin seeds

½ cup unsalted raw sunflower seeds

1. Preheat the oven to 325°F.

2. Spread the oats on a baking pan. Spread the almonds in a separate small baking pan. Place the oats and almonds in the oven and bake, stirring often, until the oats are lightly browned and the almonds are toasted. The oats will take 30 to 35 minutes; the almonds will toast in 20 to 25 minutes.

3. Place the oats and almonds in a large bowl and cool completely.

4. Add the fruit bits, wheat germ, pumpkin seeds, and sunflower seeds. Toss to combine. Store in an airtight container.

5. Serve with organic milk or yogurt.

Makes 22 servings. Per serving: *190 calories, 7 g protein, 26 g carbs, 4 g fiber, 7 g sugars, 6.5 g fat, 0 mg cholesterol, 11 mg sodium*

The *Women's Health* Diet
LUNCHES

Focus on vegetables, beans, fruits, nuts, and whole grains

Lunch is a pit stop that allows you to take on the fuel you need to power through the afternoon. Aim for at least three servings of vegetables—which are mainly water, fiber, and vitamins, so they will keep you hydrated and full with healthy calories.

Chicken and Avocado Tortilla Sandwich

1 tsp canola oil
2 corn tortillas (6" diameter)
¼ avocado, sliced
1 oz skinless chicken breast, cooked and thinly sliced
1 leaf lettuce, shredded
2 tsp store-bought salsa
2 tsp fresh cilantro, minced

1. Heat the oil in a skillet over medium-high heat. Cook the tortillas for about 1 minute on each side, or until lightly browned (they will become crisp as they cool).

2. Transfer the tortillas to a work surface. Place the avocado on 1 tortilla. Top it with the chicken, lettuce, salsa, cilantro, and remaining tortilla.

3. With a serrated knife, cut it into 2 half-moons.

Makes 1 serving. Per serving: *264.5 calories, 13 g protein, 27 g carbs, 6 g fiber, 1 g sugars, 13 g fat, 24 mg cholesterol, 112 mg sodium*

Spinach Salad with Roasted Sweet Potatoes and Warm Citrus-Ginger Dressing

2 large sweet potatoes (about 1¼ lb), peeled and cut into 1" cubes

4 Tbsp olive oil

1 tsp salt

2 thick slices bacon (2 oz total)

1 red bell pepper, chopped

1 small red onion, halved and thinly sliced

1 Tbsp fresh ginger, minced

1 tsp ground cumin

⅓ cup orange juice (1 orange)

1 lb fresh spinach leaves

   freshly ground black pepper, to taste

   pinch of salt (optional)

1. Heat oven to 400°F. Put the sweet potatoes on a baking sheet, drizzle them with 2 tablespoons of the oil, sprinkle with ¾ teaspoon of the salt, and toss to coat. Roast, turning occasionally, until crisp and brown on the outside and just tender inside, about 30 minutes. Remove them from the oven but leave them on the pan until ready to use.

2. While the potatoes roast, cook the bacon in a skillet over medium heat turning once or twice, until crisp. Drain the bacon on paper towels and pour off the fat, leaving any darkened bits in the pan. Chop the bacon. Put pan back over medium heat and add the remaining 2 tablespoons of oil. When hot, add the bell pepper, onion, ginger, and remaining ¼ teaspoon salt. Cook, stirring once or twice, until no longer raw. Stir in the cumin and bacon. Stir in the orange juice and turn off heat.

3. Put the spinach in a large bowl. Add the sweet potatoes, the warm dressing, and the freshly ground black pepper, to taste, and toss to combine. Taste and add salt if needed.

Makes 4 servings. Per serving: *274 calories, 7 g protein, 28 g carbs, 6 g fiber, 10 g sugars, 16 g fat, 4 mg cholesterol, 799 mg sodium*

Watercress Salad with Asian Pears, Smoked Trout, and Golden Beets

¾ lb golden beets, unpeeled, rinsed

2 Tbsp extra-virgin olive oil

3½ tsp lemon juice

2 tsp yuzu juice (available through gourmet Web sites, or you can use lime juice)

½ tsp salt

1 bunch watercress, thick stems trimmed

2 endives, halved lengthwise and thinly sliced crosswise

2 Asian pears, cut into ½"-thick wedges

1 (8 oz) smoked trout, skin and bones removed, cut into 8 pieces

1. Preheat the oven to 400°F. Wrap the beets in foil and place them on a baking sheet. Roast them for 1 hour and 15 minutes, or until the package yields to gentle pressure. When the beets are cool enough to handle, slip off the skins and cut them into thin wedges.

2. In a large bowl, whisk together the oil, lemon juice, yuzu juice, and salt. Add the watercress, endives, and Asian pears, and toss to coat.

3. Divide the salad among four plates and top with the beets and trout.

Makes 4 servings. Per serving: *304 calories, 22 g protein, 32.5 g carbs, 15.5 g fiber, 16 g sugars, 11 g fat, 80.5 mg cholesterol, 430 mg sodium*

Vegetarian Curry Burgers

2   Tbsp olive or canola oil

1   medium onion, chopped (about 1 cup)

1   tsp curry powder

½   tsp ground coriander

½   tsp crushed fennel seeds

1½ cups white button mushrooms, chopped

1½ cups chickpeas, cooked and drained

1   medium carrot, grated (about 1 cup)

¼   cup walnuts, chopped

3   Tbsp cilantro, chopped

½   tsp salt

¼   tsp ground black pepper flour

1. In a medium skillet over medium-high heat, warm 1 tablespoon of the oil.

2. Add the onion, curry powder, coriander, and fennel seeds. Cook, stirring frequently, for about 2 minutes, or until the onion starts to soften.

3. Add the mushrooms. Stir to mix. Cover and cook for about 4 minutes longer, or until the liquid pools in the pan.

4. Uncover and cook for about 3 minutes more, or until the liquid is evaporated.

5. Transfer the mixture to the bowl of a food processor fitted with a metal blade. Add the chickpeas. Pulse until well chopped. Transfer to a bowl.

6. Add the carrot, walnuts, cilantro, salt, and pepper to the bowl and mix well.

7. Lightly dust hands with flour. Shape the mixture into six 4"-wide patties.

8. In a large skillet over medium heat, warm the remaining 1 tablespoon of oil. Place the patties in the pan. Cook them for about 4 minutes, or until browned on the bottom. Flip them and cook for about 4 minutes longer or until heated through. Top them and serve them as you would any burger.

Makes 6 burgers. Per serving : *170 calories, 6 g protein, 18 g carbs, 5 g fiber, 4 g sugars, 9 g fat, 0 mg cholesterol, 18 mg sodium*

Slow-Cooked Pork Barbecue

1   tsp salt
1   tsp paprika
1   tsp chili powder
½   tsp ground cumin
⅛   tsp cayenne
4   lb bone-in pork shoulder, cut into 3 pieces and trimmed of all visible fat
1   onion, thinly sliced
½   cup brown sugar
½   cup ketchup
⅓   cup cider vinegar
¼   cup tomato paste
¼   cup water
2   Tbsp mustard
2   Tbsp Worcestershire sauce
½   tsp hot-pepper sauce

1. Mix the salt, paprika, chili powder, cumin, and cayenne. Rub the mixture over the pork.

2. Combine the pork and the onion, brown sugar, ketchup, cider vinegar, tomato paste, water, mustard, worcestershire sauce, and hot-pepper sauce in a large slow cooker. Cover and cook on low for 6 to 8 hours.

3. Remove the pork from the slow cooker and discard the bone. Cool for 10 minutes.

4. Using forks, shred the pork. Combine the pork with the sauce from the cooker. Serve over a toasted English muffin or hamburger bun.

Makes 12 servings. Per serving: *282 calories, 30 g protein, 14 g carbs, 1 g fiber, 13 g sugars, 11 g fat, 101 mg cholesterol, 530 mg sodium*

Grilled Fish and White Bean Salad

2 Tbsp extra-virgin olive oil
2 Tbsp lemon juice
1 tsp grated lemon zest
   pinch of coarse salt
   pinch of pepper
1½ cups skinless salmon or tuna pieces, grilled and broken into large chunks
2 cups cooked white beans
1 cup cooked green beans
1 cup grape tomatoes, halved
⅓ cup red onion, thinly sliced
1½ tsp fresh sage, thinly shredded, or rosemary leaves, minced

1. In a large bowl, whisk together the oil, lemon juice, lemon zest, salt, and pepper. Measure out 1 tablespoon of the dressing and toss it with the fish in a medium bowl.

2. In a large bowl, toss the remaining dressing with the white beans, green beans, tomatoes, onion, and sage or rosemary.

3. Divide the vegetable mixture among 4 plates and top with the fish. Serve at room temperature or chilled.

Makes 4 servings. Per serving: *374 calories, 32 g protein, 31 g carbs, 8.5 g fiber, 3 g sugars, 14 g fat, 60 mg cholesterol, 116 mg sodium*

White Bean Soup with Kale and Fresh Herbs

3   slices bacon, finely chopped
1   Tbsp olive oil
1   medium onion, finely chopped
4   cloves garlic, minced
4   cups chicken broth
4   cups cooked cannellini beans
1   small sprig fresh rosemary
1   sprig fresh sage
3   cups kale, finely chopped
    salt and pepper, to taste

1. In a heavy-bottomed soup pot, cook the bacon over medium heat until the fat has rendered and the bacon is crisp, 10 to 12 minutes. Pour off fat.

2. Add the olive oil, increase the heat to medium-high, and toss in the onion and garlic. Cook until the onion is softened and translucent, 5 to 7 minutes.

3. Add the broth, beans, rosemary, and sage and bring to a boil. Reduce the heat to medium-low and simmer for 15 minutes. Remove and discard the rosemary and sage.

4. Transfer half of the solids to a food processor or blender and combine until smooth.

5. Return the blended mixture to the soup pot and stir to combine. Bring the soup back to a quick boil, remove the pot from the heat, and add the kale. Season to taste with salt and pepper.

Makes 6 servings. Per serving: *291 calories, 18 g protein, 38 g carbs, 9 g fiber, 1 g sugars, 9 g fat, 8 mg cholesterol, 214 mg sodium*

Poached Salmon
with Honey-Mustard Vegetable Salad

2 salmon fillets (6 oz each), rinsed and dried

1 tsp dried or fresh parsley

juice of ½ lemon

1 tsp ground black pepper + 1 pinch

4 cups spinach leaves

10 grape or cherry tomatoes, halved

½ cup blueberries

1 tsp extra-virgin olive oil

½ cup sweet onion, chopped

1 clove garlic, minced

20 asparagus spears, bottoms cut off

½ yellow bell pepper, cut into strips

1 Tbsp honey mustard (use the lowest sodium one you can find)

1 Tbsp almonds, slivered

1. Place the salmon in a deep skillet big enough for the salmon to lie flat on the bottom. Cover the fish with 1" of water.

2. Add the parsley, lemon juice, and 1 teaspoon of black pepper.

3. Bring to a boil over medium heat. Boil for 10 to 15 minutes, or until the fish is opaque.

4. Lightly scrape off the skin and fat line.

5. Evenly divide the spinach, tomato, and blueberries between two plates. Top each with half of the salmon.

6. In another skillet, combine the oil, onion, and garlic. Cook over medium-high heat for 2 minutes, or until lightly browned.

7. Add the asparagus, bell pepper, and a pinch of black pepper.

8. Reduce the heat to medium. Cook for 2 to 3 minutes, or until the veggies are slightly tender.

9. Add the honey mustard. Cook for 30 seconds longer, or until the honey mustard slightly caramelizes.

10. Place the mixture over the salmon. Sprinkle with the almonds.

Makes 2 servings. Per serving: *496 calories, 42 g protein, 33 g carbs, 10 g fiber, 13 g sugars, 23 g fat, 100 mg cholesterol, 238 mg sodium*

The *Women's Health* Diet
Dinners

Focus on leafy greens and other vegetables, lean meats, fish, beans, and other legumes

Studies show that if you start your dinner with a small side salad dressed with olive oil and vinegar or with steamed folate-rich vegetables like kale, spinach, collard greens, or Swiss chard, you'll decrease your overall food intake by 12 percent while taking in satiating fiber and disease-fighting nutrients. Plus, folate-rich greens will give you a mood boost.

Grilled Mackerel with Dijon Vinaigrette

½ cup olive oil
1 Tbsp Dijon mustard
juice of 2 lemons
handful of fresh parsley
2 mackerel fillets
salt
pepper
2 cups kale

1. Whisk together the olive oil and the Dijon mustard, the lemon juice, and the parsley.

2. Season the mackerel fillets with salt and pepper and a spoonful of the vinaigrette. Cook them over medium heat on a clean, oiled grill for 3 to 4 minutes a side until they're lightly charred and firm to the touch.

3. While the fish is cooking, quickly steam the kale.

4. Combine the fish and kale and drizzle on plenty of vinaigrette before serving.

Makes 2 servings. Per serving: *347 calories, 25.5 g protein, 33 g carbs, 8 g fiber, 1 g sugars, 14 g fat, 93 mg cholesterol, 161 mg sodium*

Sage-Crusted Chicken Tenders and Crispy Kale Chips

CHICKEN TENDERS

1	egg white
1	Tbsp sesame seeds
1	Tbsp sunflower seeds, finely chopped
¾	tsp finely chopped sage
⅛	tsp freshly ground black pepper
2	boneless, skinless chicken tenders (2 oz each)
1	Tbsp spicy brown mustard
1	tsp honey

KALE CHIPS

1½	cups packed kale, cut into 1½" pieces
1	tsp garlic, minced
1	tsp extra-virgin olive oil
½	tsp sesame seeds
	salt and freshly ground pepper, to taste

1. Preheat the oven to 400°F. Coat a baking sheet with canola oil cooking spray. Place the egg white in a shallow bowl. Combine half of the sesame seeds, sunflower seeds, sage, and black pepper in another small bowl.

2. Using a fork, dip the chicken in the egg white to coat both sides, then dip them in the sesame seed mixture, coating both sides.

3. Transfer to one half of the baking sheet and mist the chicken with cooking spray. Flip the chicken with a fork and mist the other side.

4. Combine the kale, garlic, oil, and other half of the sesame seeds in a medium bowl, tossing to coat. Season with salt and freshly ground black pepper. Transfer the kale to the other half of the baking sheet. (Note: The kale does not need to be in a single layer.)

5. Bake for 15 to 17 minutes, or until the chicken is cooked through and the kale is crisp and its edges are browned. Flip the chicken and toss the kale halfway through the cooking time.

6. Combine the mustard and honey in a small bowl and serve as a dipping sauce for the chicken tenders.

Makes 1 serving. Per serving: *385 calories, 37 g protein, 22 g carbs, 4.5 g fiber, 6 g sugars, 16 g fat, 66 mg cholesterol, 324 mg sodium*

Citrus-Marinated Pork and Vegetable Fajitas

1¼ lb boneless pork loin chops, trimmed and sliced into ½" strips

grated peel and juice of 1 lime

3 cloves garlic, minced

½ tsp kosher salt

¼ tsp cayenne pepper

¼ tsp ground black pepper

4 tsp + 1 Tbsp canola oil

3 large bell peppers (mixed colors), seeded and cut into long, ½"-thick strips

1 extra-large onion, cut into ½" slices

2 jalapeño peppers, seeded and cut into thin strips

1 cup cilantro leaves, tough stems discarded and loosely packed

12 6" flour tortillas, warmed

1. Place the pork in a bowl with the lime zest, half of the lime juice, the garlic, salt, cayenne, black pepper, and 2 teaspoons of the oil. Toss to coat. Marinate the pork at room temperature for 20 minutes (or longer, or overnight in the fridge).

2. Heat 1 tablespoon of oil in a wok (or 12-inch skillet) over medium-high heat. Add the bell peppers, onion, and jalapeño. Stir-fry until the onions and peppers are soft and slightly charred, 6 to 8 minutes. Transfer the peppers and onions to a metal bowl and toss with cilantro and the remaining lime juice. Cover with foil and keep warm.

3. Return the wok to medium-high heat. Add the remaining 2 teaspoons of oil and the pork. Stir-fry until the meat is seared and just cooked through, 3 to 4 minutes. Place the pork in warmed tortillas and top with the vegetables.

Makes 6 servings. Per serving: *521 calories, 29 g protein, 58 g carbs, 5 g fiber, 6 g sugars, 19 g fat, 60 mg cholesterol, 837 mg sodium*

Pan-Sautéed Scallops with White Beans and Spinach

2   strips bacon, chopped into small pieces
½   red onion, minced
1   clove garlic, minced
1½ cans white beans (14 oz each), rinsed and drained
4   cups baby spinach
1   lb large sea scallops
    salt and pepper to taste
1   Tbsp butter
    juice of 1 lemon

1. Heat a medium saucepan on low and cook the bacon until it begins to crisp. Pour off some of the bacon fat and add the onion and garlic. Sauté until the onion is soft and translucent, about 2 to 3 minutes. Add the beans and spinach. Cook until the beans are hot and the spinach is wilted. Keep warm.

2. Heat a large cast-iron skillet or sauté pan on medium-high. Blot the scallops dry with a paper towel and season them on both sides with salt and pepper. Add the butter to the pan. After it melts, add the scallops. Sear them for 2 to 3 minutes on each side until they're deeply caramelized.

3. Before serving, add the lemon juice to the beans, along with some salt and pepper. Divide the beans among four warm bowls or plates and top them with the scallops.

Makes 4 servings. Per serving: *284 calories, 28 g protein, 28 g carbs, 7 g fiber, 2 g sugars, 7 g fat, 50 mg cholesterol, 400 mg sodium*

Black Bean & Vegetable Stir-Fry with Noodles

STIR-FRY SEASONING

2 Tbsp dried onion
2 Tbsp garlic powder
2 tsp dried parsley
½ tsp ground ginger
¼ tsp crushed red-pepper flakes
½ tsp salt

STIR-FRY

2 tsp olive oil
2 medium red bell pepper, chopped
1 small onion, chopped
1 small zucchini, halved and cut into chunks
2 cloves garlic, minced
1 bag (16 oz) shirataki noodles, drained and rinsed in hot water
1 cup canned black beans, drained and rinsed
2 Tbsp reduced-sodium soy sauce
2 Tbsp fresh cilantro, chopped hot-pepper sauce

1. In a small bowl, combine the dried onion, garlic powder, parsley, ginger, red-papper flakes, and salt.

2. Warm the oil in a wok or large cast-iron skillet over high heat. Add the bell peppers, onion, zucchini, and garlic. Reduce the heat to medium-high and cook, stirring frequently, for 4 minutes or until the vegetables start to soften.

3. Add the noodles, beans, soy sauce, and seasoning mix. Reduce the heat to medium. Cook, stirring frequently, for 3 to 4 minutes longer, or until the mixture is hot. Add the cilantro. Toss to mix.

4. Season with hot-pepper sauce to taste at the table.

Makes 4 servings. Per serving: *106.5 calories, 5 g protein, 18 g carbs, 5 g fiber, 4 g sugars, 3 g fat, 0 mg cholesterol, 538.5 mg sodium*

Sun-Dried Tomato and Feta Chicken with Spinach

2 Tbsp jarred sun-dried tomatoes, chopped

2 Tbsp feta cheese, crumbled

2 Tbsp olives, chopped

2 garlic cloves, minced

1 Tbsp balsamic vinegar

2 free-range organic chicken breasts

  extra-virgin olive oil

  salt and black pepper, to taste

2 cups organic spinach

1. Preheat the oven to 450°F. Toss together the tomatoes, feta cheese, olives, 1 clove of minced garlic, and vinegar.

2. Rub the chicken with olive oil, salt, and pepper. Using a small, sharp knife, carefully cut a slit along the thick part of each chicken breast, creating a pocket. Add enough tomato mixture to fill each pocket and transfer the chicken to a baking sheet.

3. Bake for about 15 minutes, until the chicken juices run clear. Top with any remaining stuffing.

4. While chicken is cooking, sauté the spinach with the remaining tablespoon of olive oil and minced garlic clove. Serve alongside the chicken.

Makes 2 servings. Per serving: *634 calories, 60 g protein, 29 g carbs, 2 g fiber, 4 g sugars , 29 g fat, 153 mg cholesterol, 791 mg sodium,*

Red-Lentil and Veggie Burritos

10 dry-packed sun-dried tomatoes
1 cup boiling water + 2½ cups water
1 cup dry red lentils, sorted and rinsed
1 Tbsp olive oil
½ cup onions, chopped
½ cup broccoli florets, chopped
½ cup cauliflower florets, chopped
½ cup carrots, thinly sliced
1½ cups tomato sauce
1 tsp curry powder
½ tsp ground cinnamon
4 whole-wheat tortillas (8" diameter), warmed

1. Place the sun-dried tomatoes in a small bowl and cover with the boiling water. Let soak for 10 minutes, or until the tomatoes are soft. Drain, reserving ½ cup of the soaking liquid.

2. Chop the tomatoes and set aside.

3. In a medium saucepan, combine 2½ cups of water, the lentils, and the reserved soaking liquid. Bring to a boil over medium-high heat. Reduce the heat to low and simmer for 6 to 10 minutes, or just until the lentils are tender. Drain and set aside.

4. In a large cast-iron or stainless steel skillet over medium heat, warm the oil. Add the onions, broccoli, cauliflower, and carrots. Sauté for 4 to 5 minutes or until the vegetables are tender. Stir in the tomato sauce, curry powder, and cinnamon. Add the lentils and sun-dried tomatoes. Simmer for 15 to 20 minutes, or until slightly thickened.

5. Divide the lentil mixture evenly among the tortillas. Roll and enjoy!

Makes 4 servings. Per serving: *331 calories, 19 g protein, 61 g carbs, 13 g fiber, 9 g sugars, 5 g fat, 0 mg cholesterol, 787 mg sodium*

Lemony Grilled Trout
with Fresh Herbs and Swiss Chard

2   farmed rainbow trout fillets (5 to 6 oz each)

1   lemon, thinly sliced

1   Tbsp + 2 tsp extra-virgin olive oil

sprigs of fresh basil, parsley, chervil, or lovage

kosher salt and freshly ground pepper, to taste

2   cups Swiss chard, chopped

1. Preheat the grill to medium heat, or preheat oven to 425°F. Place each fillet, skin side down, on a square of heavy-duty aluminum foil. Top each with lemon slices, 1 teaspoon of oil, and a few herb sprigs. Season lightly with salt and pepper. Fold and seal the edges of the foil to create a tent above the fillets.

2. Place packets on the grill rack (if using an oven, place on a large baking sheet) and cook, lid down, 10 to 12 minutes.

3. While the fish is cooking, sauté Swiss chard in the remaining 1 tablespoon olive oil.

4. When fish fillets are opaque, flaky, and just cooked through, remove them from heat. Let them rest for 2 minutes before serving with the chard.

Makes 2 servings. Per serving: *185 calories, 20 g protein, 1 g carbs, 0 g fiber, 0 g sugars, 11 g fat, 56 mg cholesterol, 312 mg sodium*

Maple-Dijon Pork

1   Tbsp maple syrup
1   Tbsp Dijon mustard
1   tsp olive oil
1   small clove garlic, crushed
    salt and ground black pepper, to taste
2   bone-in pork chops

1. Preheat a cast-iron skillet to medium-high.

2. In a small bowl, stir together the syrup, mustard, oil, garlic, salt, and pepper.

3. Place the pork chops and mustard mixture inside a large resealable plastic bag, then shake thoroughly to coat the chops.

4. Place the chops on the skillet, cooking 3 to 4 minutes per side. In the last minute of cooking, pour the remaining mustard mixture onto the chops.

Makes 2 servings. Per serving: *282 calories, 39 g protein, 9 g carbs, 0 g fiber, 6 g sugars, 9 g fat, 123 mg cholesterol, 575 mg sodium*

The *Women's Health* Diet
Snacks

Focus on dairy, protein, fiber-rich grains, fruit, nuts, beans, and other legumes

You can't lose weight and keep it off unless you snack! In fact, studies show that people who avoid eating between meals may end up consuming more calories overall, mostly because hungry people make bad food choices. To stay on track, choose two snacks at a time: a high-fiber carb (such as fruit) to give your brain a boost and a healthy protein or fat (like peanut butter) to help you stay satisfied longer.

Sweet and Savory Roasted Pumpkin Seeds

2 cups green pumpkin seeds
2 Tbsp pure maple syrup
1½ tsp kosher salt
½ tsp paprika or cayenne pepper

1. Preheat oven to 425°F. Toss the pumpkin seeds, syrup, salt, and paprika or cayenne together in a bowl until the seeds are well-coated.

2. Transfer the seeds and any remaining liquid to a parchment-lined baking sheet. Arrange into a single layer. Toast until the seeds are golden brown and aromatic, 10 to 15 minutes. Let cool. The seeds will keep in an airtight container at room temperature for up to 5 days.

Makes 16 servings. Per serving: *133 calories, 5 g protein, 4 g carbs, 1 g fiber, 1.5 g sugars, 11 g fat, 0 mg cholesterol, 184 mg sodium*

Chickpea and Tomato Salad

½ cup chickpeas
1 small tomato, chopped
½ Tbsp extra-virgin olive oil
juice of ½ lemon
pinch of salt
pinch of black pepper

Combine the chickpeas, tomato, olive oil, and lemon juice. Add a pinch of salt and pepper.

Makes 1 serving. Per serving: *217 calories, 8 g protein, 28 g carbs, 7.5 g fiber, 7 g sugars, 9 g fat, 0 mg cholesterol, 301.5 mg sodium*

Fruit and Almond Granola

3 cups oats
½ cup unsalted almonds, roasted
3 Tbsp whole flaxseeds
1 tsp ground cinnamon
1 cup toasted wheat germ
4 scoops vanilla whey protein powder
2 Tbsp brown sugar
3 Tbsp honey
1 cup water
3 Tbsp dried cranberries
3 Tbsp dates, chopped
2 Tbsp raisins

1. Preheat the oven to 350°F.

2. In a large bowl, mix together the oats, almonds, flaxseeds, cinnamon, wheat germ, protein powder, brown sugar, honey, and water.

3. Coat a large baking pan with cooking spray. Add the mixture and spread it from edge to edge to create an even layer.

4. Bake for 90 minutes, stirring every 15 minutes, until all the granola is browned and crunchy. If it's not crunchy after 90 minutes, bake for 15 minutes longer while watching to make sure that it doesn't get too dark.

5. Remove from the oven and allow it to cool completely.

6. Add the cranberries, dates, and raisins. Stir to mix.

Makes 7 servings. Per serving: *417 calories, 24 g protein, 57 g carbs, 9 g fiber, 23 g sugars, 12 g fat, 20 mg cholesterol, 28 mg sodium*

Tuna-Celery Sliders

1 can chunk light tuna, rinsed and drained

1 Tbsp balsamic vinegar

¼ cup onion, finely chopped

¼ cup apple, finely chopped

2 Tbsp mayonnaise

freshly ground pepper, to taste

2 celery stalks, cut into 3" pieces

1. In a bowl, mix the tuna, vinegar, onion, apple, mayonnaise, and pepper.

2. Spoon the mixture into the celery stalks, chill them for an hour or two, and enjoy.

Makes 2 servings. Per serving: *214 calories, 19 g protein, 7 g carbs, 1 g fiber, 5 g sugars, 12 g fat, 26 mg cholesterol, 160 mg sodium*

Apricots with Greek Yogurt and Honey

1 cup Greek yogurt, plain

2 Tbsp honey

½ tsp vanilla extract

6 apricots, halved lengthwise

Whisk together the yogurt, honey, and vanilla extract in small bowl. Spoon the yogurt over the apricots and serve.

Makes 2 servings. Per serving: *69 calories, 4 g protein, 13 g carbs, 1 g fiber, 12 g sugars, 1 g fat, 2 mg cholesterol, 12 mg sodium*

Toasted Almond Fruit Salad

2 Tbsp almonds, slivered and toasted

3 medium navel oranges

1 large red grapefruit

3 firm-ripe kiwifruit, peeled, ends trimmed, and cut into half-moon slices

2 Tbsp dried cherries or cranberries

1. Place the almonds in a dry cast-iron skillet over medium heat. Toast them, shaking the skillet often, for 3 to 5 minutes, or until fragrant and golden.

2. With a serrated knife, cut the skin and white pith from the oranges and grapefruit. Working over a bowl, cut in between the membranes, letting the sections drop into the bowl. Squeeze the juice from the membranes over the fruit.

3. Add the kiwi and cherries or cranberries and toss gently to mix. Spoon into bowls and top each with toasted almonds.

Makes 4 servings. Per serving: *143 calories, 3 g protein, 32 g carbs, 6 g fiber, 16 g sugars, 2 g fat, 0 mg cholesterol, 4 mg sodium*

Yogurt with Flax and Berries

½ cup mixed berries

1 tsp ground flaxseed

1 cup plain yogurt

Add the berries and flaxseed to the yogurt, mix, and enjoy!

Makes 1 serving. Per serving: *199 calories, 10 g protein, 20 g carbs, 3 g fiber, 17 g sugars, 9 g fat, 32 mg cholesterol, 114 mg sodium*

Eat a large portion
of your calories
in the morning and
you'll lose weight
and keep it off!

———————————————

Index

Boldface page references indicate photographs.
Underscored references indicate boxed text.

C

P